"Knowing is not enough; we must apply.
Willing is not enough; we must do."
—Goethe

G000069632

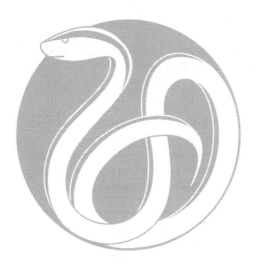

INSTITUTE OF MEDICINE

Shaping the Future for Health

THE NATIONAL ACADEMIES
National Academy of Sciences
National Academy of Engineering
Institute of Medicine
National Research Council

The **National Academy of Sciences** is a private, nonprofit, self-perpetuating society of distinguished scholars engaged in scientific and engineering research, dedicated to the furtherance of science and technology and to their use for the general welfare. Upon the authority of the charter granted to it by the Congress in 1863, the Academy has a mandate that requires it to advise the federal government on scientific and technical matters. Dr. Bruce M. Alberts is president of the National Academy of Sciences.

The **National Academy of Engineering** was established in 1964, under the charter of the National Academy of Sciences, as a parallel organization of outstanding engineers. It is autonomous in its administration and in the selection of its members, sharing with the National Academy of Sciences the responsibility for advising the federal government. The National Academy of Engineering also sponsors engineering programs aimed at meeting national needs, encourages education and research, and recognizes the superior achievements of engineers. Dr. William A. Wulf is president of the National Academy of Engineering.

The **Institute of Medicine** was established in 1970 by the National Academy of Sciences to secure the services of eminent members of appropriate professions in the examination of policy matters pertaining to the health of the public. The Institute acts under the responsibility given to the National Academy of Sciences by its congressional charter to be an adviser to the federal government and, upon its own initiative, to identify issues of medical care, research, and education. Dr. Kenneth I. Shine is president of the Institute of Medicine.

The **National Research Council** was organized by the National Academy of Sciences in 1916 to associate the broad community of science and technology with the Academy's purposes of furthering knowledge and advising the federal government. Functioning in accordance with general policies determined by the Academy, the Council has become the principal operating agency of both the National Academy of Sciences and the National Academy of Engineering in providing services to the government, the public, and the scientific and engineering communities. The Council is administered jointly by both Academies and the Institute of Medicine. Dr. Bruce M. Alberts and Dr. William A. Wulf are chairman and vice chairman, respectively, of the National Research Council.

COMMITTEE ON HIV PREVENTION STRATEGIES
IN THE UNITED STATES

HARVEY V. FINEBERG, M.D., M.P.P., Ph.D. (*Co-Chair*), Provost, Harvard University

JAMES TRUSSELL, Ph.D. (*Co-Chair*), Associate Dean and Professor of Economics and Public Affairs, Woodrow Wilson School of Public and International Affairs, Princeton University

RAYMOND BAXTER, Ph.D., Executive Vice President, The Lewin Group

WILLARD CATES, JR., M.D., M.P.H., President, Family Health International

MYRON S. COHEN, M.D., Professor of Medicine, Microbiology and Immunology; Chief, Division of Infectious Diseases; and Director, Center for Infectious Diseases, University of North Carolina at Chapel Hill

ANKE A. EHRHARDT, Ph.D., Director, HIV Center for Clinical and Behavioral Studies, New York State Psychiatric Institute, Professor of Medical Psychology, Columbia University

BRIAN FLAY, D.Phil., Professor of Community Health Sciences and Director, Health Research and Policy Centers, School of Public Health, University of Illinois at Chicago

LORETTA JEMMOTT, Ph.D., Director, Center for Urban Health Research, Associate Professor of Nursing, University of Pennsylvania

EDWARD H. KAPLAN, Ph.D., William N. and Marie A. Beach Professor of Management Sciences; Professor of Public Health, School of Management, Yale University

NANCY KASS, Sc.D., Associate Professor and Director of Program in Ethics and Health, Johns Hopkins University School of Public Health

MARSHA LILLIE-BLANTON, Dr.P.H., Vice President, Henry J. Kaiser Family Foundation

MICHAEL MERSON, M.D., Dean and Chairman of Epidemiology and Public Health, School of Medicine, Yale University

EDWARD TRAPIDO, Sc.D., Vice-Chair and Professor, Department of Epidemiology and Public Health, University of Miami

STEN H. VERMUND, M.D., Ph.D., Professor and Director, Division of Geographic Medicine, Department of Medicine; Director, Sparkman Center for International Public Health Education, School of Public Health, University of Alabama at Birmingham

v

PAUL VOLBERDING, M.D., Professor of Medicine and Director, UCSF Positive Health Program at San Francisco General Hospital; Codirector, Center for AIDS Research, University of California at San Francisco

ANDREW ZOLOPA, M.D., Assistant Professor of Medicine, School of Medicine, Stanford University; Director, Stanford Positive Care Program; and Chief, AIDS Medicine Division, Santa Clara Valley Medical Center, San Jose

EXPERT CONSULTANTS

IVAN JUZANG, M.B.A., President, MEE Productions, Philadelphia

MICHAEL A. STOTO, Ph.D., Chair and Professor of Epidemiology, George Washington University

LIAISONS FROM THE BOARD ON HEALTH PROMOTION AND DISEASE PREVENTION

JOYCE SEIKO KOBAYASHI, M.D., Director, HIV/AIDS Neuropsychiatric Consultation Services, Denver Health Medical Center

KATHLEEN E. TOOMEY, M.D., M.P.H., Director, Division of Public Health, Georgia Department of Human Resources

STAFF

MONICA S. RUIZ, Ph.D., M.P.H., Study Director

ALICIA R. GABLE, M.P.H., Research Associate

DONNA ALMARIO, Research Assistant

ANNA STATON, Project Assistant

ROSE MARIE MARTINEZ, Sc.D., Division Director

LIAISON PANEL

Federal Organizations

Judith Auerbach, Ph.D., Prevention Science Coordinator and Behavioral and Social Science Coordinator, Office of AIDS Research, National Institutes of Health

Kathy Cahill, Associate Director for Policy, Planning, and Evaluation, Office of the Director, Centers for Disease Control and Prevention

William B. Calvert, M.S., M.B.A., M.P.H., Chairman, Department of Defense Sexually Transmitted Diseases Prevention Committee and Program Manager, Sexual Health and Responsibility Program, Navy Environmental Health Center, Department of the Navy

Robert Fullilove, Ed.D., Associate Dean for Community and Minority Affairs, Columbia University School of Public Health, CDC Advisory Committee on HIV and STD Prevention

Randolph Graydon, Director, Division of Advocacy and Special Issues, Center for Medicaid and State Operations, Health Care Financing Administration

Kim Hamlett, Ph.D., Associate Director for HIV Prevention, AIDS Service, Department of Veterans Affairs

Leslie Hardy, M.H.S., Special Assistant to Assistant Secretary for Planning and Evaluation, Office of the Assistant Secretary for Planning and Evaluation, Department of Health and Human Services

King Holmes, M.D., Ph.D., Director, Center for AIDS and STD, University of Washington, CDC Advisory Committee on HIV and STD Prevention

Richard Klein, HIV/AIDS Program Director, Food and Drug Administration

Mark Magenheim, M.D., M.P.H., Medical Director, Sarasota County Health Department, CDC Advisory Committee on HIV and STD Prevention

Dorothy Mann, Southeastern Pennsylvania Family Planning Council, CDC Advisory Committee on HIV and STD Prevention

Jean McGuire, Ph.D., AIDS Director, Massachusetts Department of Public Health, AIDS Bureau, CDC Advisory Committee on HIV and STD Prevention

M. Valerie Mills, M.S.W., Associate Administrator for HIV/AIDS, Office of Policy and Program Coordination, Substance Abuse and Mental Health Services Administration

Matthew Murguia, Associate Director for Policy, White House Office of National AIDS Policy

John Palenicek, Ph.D., Director, Policy and Program Development Office, HIV/AIDS Bureau, Health Resources Services Administration

Ronald Valdiserri, M.D., M.P.H., Deputy Director, National Center for HIV, STD, and TB Prevention, Centers for Disease Control and Prevention

Deborah Von Zinkernagel, R.N., M.S., Deputy Director, Office of HIV/AIDS Policy, Office of the Secretary, U.S. Department of Health and Human Services

Captain Greg Wood, M.S.N., F.N.P., Director, Centers of Excellence, Associate Director, HIV Center of Excellence, Phoenix Medical Center, Indian Health Service, United States Public Health Service

State and Local Organizations

Guthrie Birkhead, M.D., M.P.H., Director, AIDS Institute, New York Department of Health, Council of State and Territorial Epidemiologists

Joe Cronauer, Co-Director, AIDS Activities Coordinating Office, Philadelphia Department of Public Health, National Association of County and City Health Officials

Helen Fox-Fields, Senior Director for Infectious Disease Policy, Association of State and Territorial Health Officers

Martin Gonzales-Rojas, CDC Community Planning Group, Chicago, Illinois

David Johnson, M.D., M.P.H., Deputy Director for Public Health and Chief Medical Executive, Michigan Department of Community Health, Association of State and Territorial Health Officers

Leigh Lipson, Program Associate, National Association of County and City Health Officials

John Middaugh, M.D., Alaska State Epidemiologist, Council of State and Territorial Epidemiologists

Julie Scofield, Executive Director, National Alliance of State and Territorial AIDS Directors

Evelyn Ullah, B.S.N., M.S.W., Director, Office of HIV/AIDS Services, Miami-Dade County Health Department, Miami Crisis Response Team Liaison, Congressional Black Caucus Initiative

Nongovernmental Organizations

Larry Abrams, Associate Director of Prevention, Gay Men's Health Crisis

Julio Abreu, Associate Director of Government Affairs, AIDS Action Council

Terje Anderson, Executive Director, National Association of People with AIDS

Cornelius Baker, Executive Director, Whitman Walker Clinic

Ignatius Bau, J.D., Policy Director, Asian and Pacific Islander American Health Forum

Lorraine Cole, Ph.D., Executive Director, National Medical Association

Blake Cornish, Federal Legislative Lawyer, National Gay/Lesbian Task Force

Lawrence D'Angelo, M.D., M.P.H, Society for Adolescent Medicine

Debra Fraser-Howze, Chief Executive Officer, The National Black Leadership Commission on AIDS

Leroy Gross, M.D., M.P.H., Aerospace Medicine Regent, American College of Preventive Medicine

Christopher La Bonte, Senior Policy Advocate, Human Rights Campaign

Miguelina Ileana León, Director of Government Relations and Public Policy, National Minority AIDS Council

Barbara Menard, Senior Policy Advocate, Human Rights Campaign Commission on AIDS

Wayne J. Mitchell, Ph.D., Executive Director, Association for Drug Abuse Treatment and Prevention

Clark Moore, Director for Policy and Communications, AIDS Alliance for Children, Youth, and Families

Martin Ornelas-Quintero, Executive Director, The National Latina/Latino Lesbian, Gay, Bisexual, and Transgender Organization

Sally Raphel, M.S., R.N., Director of Nursing Practice, American Nurses Association

Elena Rios, President, Hispanic Medical Association

Ron Rowell, M.P.H., Executive Director, National Native American AIDS Prevention Center

Jane Silver, Director of Public Policy, American Foundation for AIDS Research

Shepherd Smith, President, Children's AIDS Fund

Research Institutions

Thomas Coates, Ph.D., Director, Center for AIDS Prevention Studies, University of California at San Francisco

James Curran, M.D., M.P.H, Dean, Rollins School of Public Health, Director, Center for AIDS Research, Emory University

Robert H. Remien, Ph.D., Research Scientist, HIV Center for Clinical and Behavioral Studies, New York State Psychiatric Institute and Columbia University

Preface

Through 1999, more than 733,000 acquired immune deficiency syndrome (AIDS) cases and 430,000 deaths from human immunodeficiency virus (HIV) infection and AIDS have been reported in the United States. Prevention efforts conducted by federal, state, and local government agencies, nongovernmental organizations, and the private sector have shown considerable success in slowing the rapid growth of the epidemic. However, the demographic face of the epidemic is changing dramatically; this in turn, is changing how the nation must respond. Men who have sex with men remain at high risk in many areas. However, racial and ethnic minorities, women, adolescents, and young adults are increasingly affected by HIV/AIDS. In addition, recent improvements in the treatment of HIV disease have enabled more people to live longer with HIV and AIDS, but have contributed to a growing complacency toward the disease. The promise of a vaccine for HIV remains only a hope, not a reality.

Given these challenges, the Centers for Disease Control and Prevention (CDC) requested that the Institute of Medicine convene a committee to conduct a comprehensive review of current HIV prevention efforts in the United States. Specifically, this Committee on HIV Prevention Strategies in the United States was asked to review the HIV prevention efforts of the CDC and other Department of Health and Human Services (DHHS) agencies, as well as the efforts of various other public and private sector agencies and organizations, and to examine the changing nature of the epidemic, advances in clinical prevention and treatment, evaluations of public health interventions, and emerging research in the behavioral sciences and its impact on HIV prevention. Based on this review, the Committee was asked to propose a visionary framework for future national HIV prevention activities and suggest institutional roles for the CDC and other federal, public, and private sector agencies in the context of this framework.

The Committee met four times over a 5-month period between January and May 2000. During this time, we held three workshops with a variety of federal agencies, state and local organizations, nongovernmental organizations, and researchers regarding current HIV prevention activities. The Committee engaged in several additional data gathering activities to gain input regarding HIV prevention efforts at the federal, state, and local levels. These activities included site visits to several state health departments, a site visit to the Community Planning Leadership Summit conference in Los Angeles, and a request for public comment. The Committee also reviewed the current literature and received a significant amount of information from our liaison panel, which was comprised of representatives of federal, state and local agencies and organizations, as well as of advocacy and research organizations (listed on pages *vii–ix*). Based on this evidence, the Committee identified the fundamental components of a visionary framework for a national HIV prevention strategy. These components are described and explained in the subsequent chapters of this report.

Given the broad scope of the Committee's charge, the complexity of the issues, and the limited time allowed for conducting the work and writing the report (seven months), we made several important decisions regarding how we would approach the task. First, the Committee chose to focus on a framework of principles to guide future HIV prevention efforts, rather than to develop a detailed road map for conducting HIV prevention activities. Second, the Committee chose as a starting point for this framework the principle that the nation should have an explicit prevention goal: **to avert as many new HIV infections as possible with the resources available for HIV prevention.** While this may seem an obvious goal, we found that many current HIV prevention efforts are inconsistent with this principle.

The Committee recognized that there are a number of factors that can undermine public health goals, including those related to HIV prevention:

- inappropriate considerations are used to frame policy choices;

- suboptimal decision rules are applied to the problem;
- social values and prejudices do not support the policy goal;
- insufficient resources hinder the successful implementation of the policy goal;
- organizational or structural factors impede implementation of policies;
- failures in implementation, related to such factors as inadequate training or lack of operating capacity, detract from the desired outcome of averting new infections.

In light of the Committee's limited time frame and our desire to provide a guiding framework, we chose to focus on the first three factors: framing HIV prevention policy choices, decision making for allocating federal prevention funds, and overcoming social obstacles to success.

The Committee's visionary framework for HIV prevention suggests new directions for HIV/AIDS surveillance, resource allocation, the incorporation of prevention into the clinical setting, technology development, and the translation of research into practice. We also discuss the social and political barriers that continue to limit the success of HIV prevention. Although many of these barriers have been addressed in previous Institute of Medicine and other public health reports, the Committee felt it would be unconscionable not to restate its opposition to these powerful forces that have impeded prevention efforts.

The Committee is aware that in providing this set of principles to guide future HIV prevention activities, several aspects of the framework will require the gathering and application of better data, as well as the development of closer working relationships between federal, state, and local agencies, before recommendations can be fully implemented. We nevertheless, believe that these factors do not detract from the importance of a sound foundation for decision making. It simply means that the organizations and institutions involved in HIV prevention should work toward these goals using the best available data while seeking sounder data with which to better inform future decisions.

While the Committee observed ample evidence of the lack of federal leadership in HIV prevention, we do not focus on this issue in this report. Today, many different agencies share responsibility for federal HIV prevention activities (see Appendix C), and sometimes compete for resources and public attention.

While federal officials and agencies have tried several different leadership models to better coordinate and lead HIV prevention efforts, none has yet been very effective in bringing about the type of overarching guidance that is needed to coordinate federal prevention agencies and activities, as well as to bring together the wide variety of DHHS, non-DHHS, and outside constituencies that are involved in HIV prevention efforts. Previous studies have examined these issues and made recommendations to resolve interagency[1] and intra-agency[2] coordination and leadership problems. The Committee joins these panels and others in calling for a unified framework for managing federal HIV prevention activities. Reclaiming federal leadership of the nation's HIV prevention strategy requires better coordination of efforts that are currently too dispersed.

Additionally, the Committee's charge was limited to examining HIV prevention efforts in the United States. However, we believe that significant attention must also be directed to improving HIV prevention efforts at the global level, and to doing more to ameliorate the devastating impact that HIV/AIDS has had on the health and social and economic welfare of developing nations.

The Committee has been motivated by the conviction that the nation can and should do more to prevent HIV infection, and that the efforts to bring these objectives to fruition must begin now. The past two decades of HIV prevention activities are a testament to the fact that prevention is effective. And, given the social complacency that has emerged along with the recent therapeutic advances in HIV treatment, prevention will be even more important in the decades to come. The Committee believes that there is still much to be done, and that the successful experiences of other countries' HIV prevention efforts—particularly those demonstrating the critical importance of political leadership and commitment, community mobilization, and the removal of social barriers—provide some valuable "lessons learned" for future HIV prevention activities in the United States. Given this, the Committee remains firm in our conviction that the nation, working in a coordinated manner and with due haste, can do more to slow and perhaps even halt the spread of this deadly epidemic.

Harvey V. Fineberg, *Cochair*
James Trussell, *Cochair*

---

[1]The 1994 report to then Assistant Secretary of Health, Philip Lee, made strong recommendations aimed at resolving many of the coordination and leadership issues regarding HIV prevention within the Department of Health and Human Services (DHHS, 1994).

[2]The 1999 review of CDC's HIV/AIDS activities by the CDC Advisory Council on HIV Prevention identified opportunities for improved programmatic and budgetary coordination within the agency (CDC Advisory Committee, 1999).

REFERENCES

Centers for Disease Control and Prevention Advisory Committee for HIV and STD Prevention (CDC Advisory Committee). 1999. Work Group Report on HIV Prevention Activities at the CDC.

Department of Health and Human Services, Coordinating Group on HIV/AIDS (DHHS). 1994. HIV Prevention Work Group Recommendations, report to Philip Lee and Patsy Fleming. Washington, DC: DHHS.

Acknowledgments

This report represents the collaborative efforts of many organizations and individuals, without whom this study would not have been possible. The Committee extends its most sincere gratitude to the organizations and individuals mentioned below.

Numerous individuals and organizations generously shared their knowledge and expertise with the Committee through their active participation in Committee workshops that were held on January 23, March 1–2, and April 13, 2000. These sessions were intended to gather information related to current HIV prevention activities in order to help inform the Committee's vision of future prevention efforts. These individuals are listed in Appendix F.

Members of the study's liaison panel contributed valuable information and suggestions that were helpful in preparing this report. These organizations and their representatives to the liaison panel are listed on pages *vii–ix*.

The directors and staff of the Colorado, Maryland, New York, and Connecticut state health departments hosted individual committee members during site visits. Additionally, the Centers for Disease Control and Prevention hosted the project staff during a site visit to its main offices in Atlanta, GA.

The Committee would like to thank all of the individuals at the Community Planning and Leadership Summit in Los Angeles, CA, on March 29–31, 2000, who discussed the current state of HIV prevention and shared their experiences in conducting HIV prevention at the state, local, and community level with us. Julie Scofield, Executive Director of the National Association of State and Territorial AIDS Directors, was instrumental in facilitating the Committee's public hearing and focus groups at this meeting. The Committee is grateful to all of the individuals who shared their experiences via their responses to the Committee's request for public comment.

The Committee would like to thank the numerous staff members of the Institute of Medicine, the National Research Council, and the National Academy Press who contributed to the development, production, and dissemination of this report. The Committee is most grateful to Monica Ruiz who did a remarkable job of directing a very fast-track, complex, and demanding study, and to Alicia Gable, who showed exceptional skill in conducting research and assisting in project management. Donna Almario provided outstanding research support, as well as guidance to the new staff on IOM procedures. Cara Christie provided excellent administrative support through the first three months of the study. Anna Staton was an invaluable project assistant, who skillfully coordinated Committee meetings, organized site visits, and maintained project records and files. Rose Martinez and Susanne Stoiber provided guidance and assistance above and beyond the call of duty. Kathleen Stratton and Donna Duncan provided valuable support and advice regarding project organization. Andrea Cohen and Melissa Goodwin handled the financial accounting of the study. Mike Edington provided editorial assistance. Jennifer Otten, Vanee Vines, Neil Tickner, Jim Jensen, and Sandra McDermin provided assistance with report dissemination. We are especially grateful to Claudia Carl and Clyde Behney for cheerfully and skillfully guiding the staff through the report review process.

In addition to IOM staff, we are most grateful to Jennifer Rubin for her assistance in preparing the data needed for the resource allocation scenarios in Chapter 3, to Jeffrey Levi and Andy Schneider for their noteworthy contributions to Chapter 4, and to Tom Burroughs for invaluable assistance in drafting appendices and editing the report.

The Centers for Disease Control and Prevention generously provided funding and lent support to this project. Our project liaisons—Ronald Valdiserri, Lydia Ogden, and Eva Margolies Seiler—were extraordinarily helpful in providing data, information, and support throughout the course of the study. Their encouragement and support are gratefully acknowledged.

REVIEWERS

The report was reviewed by individuals chosen for their diverse perspectives and technical expertise in accordance with procedures approved by the National Research Council's Report Review Committee. The purpose of this independent review is to provide candid and critical comments to assist the authors and the Institute of Medicine in making the report as sound as possible and to ensure that the report meets institutional standards for objectivity, evidence, and responsiveness to the study charge. The content of the review comments and the draft manuscript remain confidential to protect the integrity of the deliberative process. The Committee wishes to thank the following individuals for their participation in the report review process:

Karen Basen-Engquist, Ph.D., Department of Behavioral Science, The University of Texas, M.D. Anderson Cancer Center, Houston
Ronald Bayer, Ph.D., Columbia University School of Public Health
Sophia Chang, M.D., M.P.H., Director, Center for Quality Management in HIV Care, Department of Veterans Affairs, Palo Alto, California
Thomas Coates, Ph.D., Director, Center for AIDS Prevention Studies, University of California at San Francisco
Gerald Friedland, M.D., Director, Yale AIDS Program, Yale University School of Medicine
James O. Kahn, M.D., Positive Health Program, San Franciso General Hospital
Harold Pollack, Ph.D., Department of Health Management and Policy, University of Michigan
Liza Solomon, Dr.P.H., Director, Maryland State AIDS Administration
Darrell P. Wheeler, Ph.D., Assistant Professor, Columbia University School of Social Work

Although the reviewers listed above have provided many constructive comments and suggestions, they were not asked to endorse the conclusions or recommendations nor did they see the final draft of the report before its release. The review of this report was overseen by Kristine M. Gebbie, Dr.P.H., R.N., Associate Professor of Nursing, Columbia University, appointed by the Institute of Medicine and Charles C.J. Carpenter, M.D., Professor of Medicine, The Miriam Hospital, Brown University, appointed by the NRC's Report Review Committee, who were responsible for making certain that an independent examination of this report was carried out in accordance with institutional procedures and that all review comments were carefully considered. Responsibility for the final content of this report rests entirely with the authoring committee and the institution.

Contents

No Time To Lose

Getting More from
HIV Prevention

Executive Summary

T wo decades after the first case of the acquired immunodeficiency syndrome (AIDS) was recognized in the United States, the nation does not have a comprehensive, effective, and efficient strategy for preventing the spread of the human immunodeficiency virus (HIV). The need for such a plan is becoming even more pressing as, ironically, advances in treating AIDS have helped foster a growing sense of complacency in many sectors of both the government and the general public, as well as in some populations of HIV-infected persons and those at high risk of becoming infected. Improved treatment is critically important, and efforts should be continued to extend such advances. With better treatment, more Americans are living with HIV/AIDS than ever before. However, this creates more opportunities for transmitting the virus and thus a greater need for prevention. Therefore, it is time for the nation to adopt a coordinated set of strategies to prevent the spread of HIV/AIDS. We must learn from our past successes, as well as from our failures, in prevention and we must focus prevention efforts on those individuals and communities who are increasingly affected by the epidemic.

By the end of 1999, a total of 733,374 AIDS cases and 430,411 AIDS-related deaths had been reported in the United States (CDC, 2000a). During the first decade of the epidemic, the number of new AIDS cases increased by 65–90 percent each year (CDC, 1996). In 1996, the number of new AIDS cases and deaths fell for the first time in the history of the epidemic (CDC, 1997). By 1998, the number of AIDS deaths had declined by almost two-thirds from the 1995 record high (CDC, 2000a). These de-

1

clines can be attributed to advances in antiretroviral therapies (CDC, 1999a) and, in part, to a number of HIV prevention efforts carried out by federal, state, and local government agencies, nonprofit organizations, and the private sector. Most notable were prevention efforts that led to: changes in sexual behavior among men who have sex with men, reduced transmission among injection drug users, increased safety of the nation's blood supply, and reduced perinatal transmission from infected mothers to their children. Recent data suggest that the declining trends in AIDS incidence and deaths may be stabilizing, however (CDC, 2000b).

Despite the enormous successes in HIV prevention over the past decade, there are additional prevention challenges. The populations that need to be reached by prevention interventions have changed considerably. Women, youth, and racial and ethnic minorities now account for a growing proportion of new AIDS cases, and increasing numbers of cases are emerging in rural and smaller urban areas (CDC, 2000a), whereas many prevention programs have previously focused on gay white men in major metropolitan areas. In addition, an increasing proportion of new AIDS cases are now being linked to heterosexual exposure, while a declining proportion of new cases are being attributed to men who have sex with men. Men who have sex with men still remain the largest exposure group, however (CDC, 2000a). These new at-risk populations are not being reached for prevention as effectively, or on as large a scale, as at-risk populations have been in the past, and prevention programs tailored to specific social contexts of an earlier period in the epidemic are not proving as effective during the current period.

As a result of such challenges, the Centers for Disease Control and Prevention requested that the Institute of Medicine convene a committee to review current HIV prevention efforts in the United States, to develop a visionary framework for a national HIV prevention strategy that could significantly reduce new infections, and to suggest the roles that public and private-sector agencies should have within this framework. The Committee examined the available evidence, and received much useful information and advice from federal, state, and local agencies, as well as from community organizations involved in research on HIV prevention and in implementing HIV prevention programs. The Committee's review revealed several important findings.

Above all, HIV prevention works: there is a wide range of proven strategies to reduce behaviors that increase the risk of transmitting or acquiring HIV. However, the ways in which prevention efforts are currently being implemented do not allow the nation to fully reap the benefits of these proven strategies. The Committee identified a number of problems.

First, expenditures on HIV prevention activities appear to be allocated to states in rough proportion to the distribution of persons with AIDS. While this approach may be useful for allocating funds for treatment, it is an inadequate marker of need for prevention services. Second, due to long-standing concerns about AIDS-related stigma and discrimination, prevention efforts have largely avoided interventions directed at individuals who are HIV-infected, the very persons who are in a unique position to stop the spread of HIV. Third, community organizations that try to conduct prevention programs are often hampered by inadequate dissemination of state-of-the-art prevention research and limited technical assistance for program adaptation, implementation, and evaluation. Fourth, neither the public nor the private sector has invested sufficiently in developing new biomedical tools and technologies that can help in HIV prevention. Finally, social barriers, such as poverty, racism, gender inequality, and the stigma attached to HIV and AIDS, continue to seriously impede HIV prevention efforts.*

The Committee also found that there is a definite lack of federal leadership with regard to HIV prevention. While the Committee does not focus in this report on the role of federal leadership, we are well aware that there have been longstanding problems related to such issues as agency organizational and structural factors and the lack of intra- and interagency coordination. Many different agencies now share responsibility for federal HIV prevention activities (see Appendix C). These agencies are funded through different sources, serve different constituents, have programmatic responsibilities other than HIV, and report to different congressional oversight and appropriations committees. Sometimes these agencies compete for resources and public attention. While federal agencies and officials have tried several different leadership models, none has been very effective in bringing about the type of overarching guidance needed to coordinate federal prevention agencies and activities, as well as to bring together the wide variety of DHHS, non-DHHS, and outside agencies that are involved in HIV prevention efforts. Reclaiming federal leadership of the nation's HIV prevention strategy requires better coordination of efforts currently too dispersed. The implementation of even the best prevention strategy will not be fully effective under conditions of poor leadership and inadequate political commitment. The Committee believes that, for HIV prevention efforts to have maximum impact, there

---

*Although the Committee's charge was limited to examining and providing a visionary framework for HIV prevention in the United States, significant attention must also be directed to improving HIV prevention efforts at the global level and to ameliorating the devastating impact that HIV/AIDS has had in developing nations.

must be a strong, clear leadership structure in the Department of Health and Human Services.

From these findings, the Committee recommends a new strategy for preventing HIV infections. As a starting point, the nation should adopt an explicit prevention goal: **to avert as many new HIV infections as possible with the resources available for HIV prevention.** While this may seem an obvious goal, the Committee found that many current HIV prevention efforts are inconsistent with this principle. To reach this goal, a new vision is needed that will improve the way the epidemic is monitored, change how prevention resources are allocated and how activities are prioritized and conducted, foster interactions between the public and private sectors to promote new prevention tools and technologies, and reduce or eliminate social barriers to HIV prevention.

This strategic vision is comprised of six elements:

- develop an accurate surveillance system, focused on new HIV infections, that can better predict where the epidemic is headed;
- allocate prevention resources to prevent as many new HIV infections as possible, guided by principles of cost-effectiveness rather than simply by the number of AIDS cases;
- direct prevention services to HIV-infected persons, who often have been excluded from prevention activities, and integrate prevention activities into the clinical setting in order to reach people at high risk of becoming infected;
- translate findings from prevention research into action at the community level;
- invest in the development of new tools and technologies to expand HIV prevention efforts; and
- strive to overcome social barriers and to remove policy barriers that impede HIV prevention.

DEVELOPING AN ACCURATE SURVEILLANCE SYSTEM FOCUSED ON NEW HIV INFECTIONS

To best plan and evaluate prevention activities and allocate resources for HIV prevention, a national surveillance system is needed that identifies new HIV infections (HIV incidence). The current epidemiological surveillance system—which is based primarily on AIDS case reporting and, more recently, on HIV case reporting in selected states—does not provide a complete or accurate picture of HIV incidence. By focusing mainly on AIDS cases, where diagnosis lags approximately 10 years after HIV infection without treatment and even longer than 10 years with potent new antiretroviral therapies, today's surveillance system looks at the past rather than to the future. The system tracks where the epidemic has been rather than where it is going. This lag is particularly problematic in light of the reality that the epidemic has shifted into new population groups. Thus, to more effectively direct prevention interventions to communities at risk, the Committee recommends that:

> **The Centers for Disease Control and Prevention create a surveillance system that can provide national population-based estimates of HIV incidence. The recommended surveillance system would estimate new HIV infections using blinded serosurveys of well-characterized sentinel populations (e.g., drug users in treatment, people attending sexually transmitted disease clinics and tuberculosis clinics, clinics serving women of reproductive age), surveys that characterize the populations served by those sites, and advanced testing technologies that are able to identify recent HIV infections.**

ALLOCATING RESOURCES TO PREVENT AS MANY NEW HIV INFECTIONS AS POSSIBLE

The current distribution of federal funds for HIV prevention can best be described as an amalgam of administrative and legislative decisions that have been shaped in response to available data, congressional mandates and earmarks, constituency pressures, personal values, and the professional judgment of program managers. The allocation strategy that results from these cumulative decisions can best be described as "proportionality." As a prevention strategy, proportionality has one important advantage in that it begins with an objective criterion of need—that is, observed AIDS cases. However, proportionality has serious limitations, including the fact that it is an inadequate marker of need for the purposes of prevention. Proportionality rewards the reporting of AIDS cases rather than the prevention of new infections. Also, current funding decisions too often ignore the cost-effectiveness of interventions, and agencies that fund prevention research activities often fall short of requiring (and funding) assessments of the cost-effectiveness of programs or interventions tested. The Committee believes that in order to avert as many new infections as possible, better decisions about the overall investment of prevention resources must be made. To this end, the Committee recommends a strategy of allocating funds based on HIV incidence and the use of cost-effective interventions. Directing prevention efforts to populations at high risk of infection, and using interventions of proven efficacy and cost-effectiveness, could prevent an estimated 20 percent to 30 percent more infections than does the current allocation of HIV prevention funds (see Chapter 3). Thus, the Committee recommends that:

Prevention resources should be allocated to prevent as many new infections as possible. Such an allocation must take into account the cost and effectiveness of programs, in addition to estimates of HIV incidence. Evaluation should be a major component of resource allocation decisionmaking. With better evaluation data reflecting the cost, efficacy, and reach of programs, resources could be more profitably invested in interventions that work. Interventions that do not work, or that are very expensive relative to the number of infections prevented, could be abandoned.

USING THE CLINICAL SETTING FOR PREVENTION

Every new HIV infection begins with someone who is already infected—yet current prevention programs do not emphasize directing prevention efforts to individuals who are HIV-infected and who may still engage in risky behavior. Ideally, prevention interventions should be available for all HIV-infected persons. According to recent data, the majority of HIV-infected persons who know their status are in the treatment system (Bozzette et al., 1998) and may receive at least some information about prevention. However, it is estimated that up to one-third of infected persons do not know their HIV status (CDC, 1999b). Efforts should be made to increase the number of infected individuals who are aware of their status. In addition, individuals at high risk for HIV infection often come in contact with the health care system for services at a variety of different entry points, and each of these clinical settings provides valuable opportunities for delivering HIV prevention services. Thus, the Committee recommends that:

> Prevention services for HIV-infected persons should be a standard of care in all clinical settings (e.g., primary care centers, sexually transmitted diseases clinics, drug treatment facilities, and mental health centers). Health care providers should have adequate training, time, and resources to conduct effective HIV prevention counseling. Enabling this activity may require adjustments in health care provider time allocations and/or specific financial incentives from public and private sources of health coverage.

TRANSLATING RESEARCH INTO ACTION

Limited information is available on the performance and cost-effectiveness of prevention programs when implemented in community settings under nonexperimental conditions. This type of information is needed to ensure that programs of proven efficacy achieve maximum possible effectiveness and cost-effectiveness once integrated into practice, to ensure that sound evaluation data are available at the community level, and to ensure that effective prevention programs are translated and disseminated into communities. As a result, the Committee recommends that:

> **Key Department of Health and Human Services agencies that fund HIV prevention research and interventions should invest in strengthening local-level capacity to develop, evaluate, implement, and support effective programs in the community. The Committee further recommends that these agencies invest in research on how best to adapt effective programs for use in community-level interventions and research on what constitutes effective technical assistance for optimal research-to-community transfer of prevention programs; these agencies should also be responsible for the widespread dissemination of the results of this research. Such efforts will require the participation and collaboration of the funding agencies, researchers, service providers, and communities.**

INVESTING IN THE DEVELOPMENT OF NEW TOOLS AND TECHNOLOGIES FOR HIV PREVENTION

Given the success that technologies have had in preventing HIV—such as antibody tests used to screen the blood supply, and drugs to prevent perinatal transmission of HIV—investment in new tools and technologies is clearly warranted. Research and product advances in the areas of HIV vaccines, antiretroviral and antimicrobial therapy, microbicides, and barrier methods (female condoms) can significantly increase the effectiveness of HIV prevention efforts. However, there are significant barriers to development, approval, and distribution of technological innovations. Such barriers include insufficient funding to maintain research on product development and testing, as well as lack of interest in the development of specific products. The timely development of new products will require the promotion of public and private sector collaborations and the development of incentives to increase involvement by private sector industries and philanthropic sources. Thus, the Committee recommends that:

> **Federal agencies should continue to invest in the development of products and technologies linked to HIV prevention. In par-**

ticular, the National Institutes of Health should place high priority on the development of anti-HIV microbicides and vaccines, and this prioritization should be accompanied by increases in funding. Similarly, the Food and Drug Administration should accelerate its efforts to approve prevention technologies that show promise in clinical trials (e.g., new antiretroviral therapies, new microbicidal and vaccine candidates) or are already being successfully utilized elsewhere in the world (e.g., rapid testing assays other than the Single Use Diagnostic System [SUDS]). For all new prevention tools, investigations of cost-effectiveness and user acceptability should be included as part of the research agenda. Federal agencies should also seek to develop stronger research collaborations with private industry, and they should offer incentives to encourage private industry investment.

STRIVING TO OVERCOME SOCIAL BARRIERS

Social, economic, and cultural forces not only shape the progression and course of the AIDS epidemic but also influence this nation's response to the epidemic. Societal attitudes surrounding sexual activity and drug use have fostered policies that have created barriers to the implementation of proven HIV prevention interventions and the efficient use of prevention resources. The consequence is missed opportunities to prevent new HIV infections, resulting in lost lives and wasted expenditures. National leadership is urgently needed to provide a coordinated strategy for effectively overcoming these social barriers in order to capitalize on the unrealized opportunities in HIV prevention. Thus, the Committee recommends:

- increasing drug abuse treatment funding to levels that are sufficient to provide drug treatment to all those requesting it;
- removing legal and policy barriers that limit access to sterile drug injection equipment;
- eliminating congressional, federal, state, and local requirements that public funds be used for abstinence-only education, and that states and local school districts implement and continue to support age-appropriate comprehensive sex education and condom availability programs in schools; and
- removing policy barriers that hinder the implementation of effective prevention efforts in correctional settings.

The Committee believes the nation can and should do more to prevent HIV infection—and we have no time to lose. Doing better will require a new way of thinking about cost-effectiveness as a guiding principle for HIV prevention. It will require new leadership, accountability, and coordination. It will require directing interventions to those who are HIV-infected and to those—the women, youth, and racial and ethnic minorities—who are increasingly affected by the epidemic. It will require more effective translation of interventions that prevent HIV in research settings into activities that are effective in communities. And it will require removing obstacles that impede the implementation of those interventions that we now know to be effective.

REFERENCES

Bozzette SA, Berry SH, Duan N, Frankel MR, Leibowitz AA, Lefkowitz D, Emmons CA, Senterfitt JW, Berk ML, Morton SC, Shapiro MF. 1998. The care of HIV-infected adults in the United States. HIV Cost and Services Utilization Study Consortium. *New England Journal of Medicine* 339(26):1897–1904.

Centers for Disease Control and Prevention. (CDC). 2000a. HIV/AIDS Surveillance Report, 1999 11(2).

Centers for Disease Control and Prevention (CDC). 2000b. U.S. AIDS Cases, Deaths, and HIV Infections Appear Stable. AMA Press Briefing, July 8.

Centers for Disease Control and Prevention. (CDC). 1999a. HIV/AIDS Surveillance Report, Mid-year 1999 11(1).

Centers for Disease Control and Prevention. (CDC). 1999b. Statistical Projections. Available on line at: www.cdc.gov/hiv/hivinfo/vfax/260210.htm

Centers for Disease Control and Prevention (CDC). 1997. Update: Trends in AIDS incidence—United States, 1996. *Morbidity and Mortality Weekly Report* 46:861–867.

Centers for Disease Control and Prevention. (CDC). 1996. 1996 HIV/AIDS Trends Provide Evidence of Success in HIV Prevention and Treatment.

1

Introduction:
Rethinking HIV Prevention

At the request of the U.S. Centers for Disease Control and Prevention (CDC), the Committee examined current HIV prevention efforts in the United States, with the objective of devising a sound framework for a national HIV prevention strategy and suggesting institutional roles within this framework for the CDC and other public and private-sector agencies. Our examination yielded three firm conclusions. First, prevention works. The nation needs to focus on strategies proven to reduce behaviors (such as having unprotected sex or sharing drug injection equipment) that risk transmitting or acquiring HIV. Such strategies are especially important because an effective HIV vaccine is not likely to be available in the near future. Second, by better allocating available funds, even more HIV infections could be averted. Third, social forces and risky behaviors fuel the spread of HIV. Poverty, racism, homophobia, and the stigma attached to HIV infection and AIDS seriously impede HIV prevention efforts. The Committee's reasons for reaching these conclusions, and a set of recommendations, follow in the substantive chapters of this report. In this introduction, we briefly justify these key findings and the implications that flow from them.

The Committee adopted the principle that the explicit goal of a national strategy should be *to avert as many new HIV infections as possible with the resources available for prevention.* One implication of this proposed goal is that HIV prevention activities will be most successful if they are directed at the persons most likely to transmit or acquire HIV—that is, those who have unprotected sex or who share drug injection equipment with persons who are HIV-infected. Increasingly, in this country, those at high risk are women, youth, and racial and ethnic minorities. While this priority may seem logical, however past HIV prevention activities have not focused on HIV-infected persons because of concerns about increased discrimination, prejudice, and the stigma associated with HIV/AIDS. While these concerns are still valid, the benefits of antiretroviral treatments, the growing evidence of ongoing risk behaviors in identified infected persons, and the need to access infected individuals in confidential and professional health care settings compels their inclusion in prevention efforts. However, directing prevention efforts to those who are infected and monitoring the course of the epidemic requires an effective HIV surveillance system, which currently does not exist.

Additionally, federal expenditures on HIV prevention activities appear to be allocated to states in rough proportion to the distribution of persons with AIDS. Indeed, achieving such a proportional allocation appears to be the current goal. If we were considering HIV treatment, then this basis for distributing resources would be reasonable. However, such a distribution model does not prevent the maximum number of new infections; it ignores the differential cost of preventing new infections across prevention activities, and it uses inappropriate data (i.e., AIDS surveillance) to make resource allocations for more current HIV incidence-driven needs.

HIV prevention efforts also must be selected with more attention given to cost-effectiveness. Not only did the Committee find that there is limited information on the cost-effectiveness of current prevention strategies, but we also discovered that virtually none of the actors in HIV prevention at the federal, state, and local levels even thinks about cost-effectiveness as a guiding principle. The Committee acknowledges that cost-effectiveness alone is insufficient as a determinant of resource allocation, since such matters as fairness and equity also deserve consideration. The nation may decide to spend some HIV prevention dollars on a particular group, even if this results in fewer infections prevented overall. But in doing so, the cost of such a decision, in terms of forgone infections prevented, should be clearly acknowledged.

Finally, the Committee was struck by how severely social barriers still deter HIV prevention. For example, the nation is spending approximately $440 million in federal and state funds over five years on abstinence-only sex education—in the absence of any evidence that this approach is effective, much less cost-effective—solely because of social forces that prevent effective comprehensive sex education courses from being offered. Further, in an effort to make the blood supply as safe as possible, the nation has spent $60 million to prevent an estimated eight new infections, or $7.5 million for each infection prevented. Yet, the federal government bars its funds from being spent to ensure drug users access to sterile drug injection equipment, a highly cost-effective prevention strategy for those who are at high risk of acquiring HIV because they use injectable drugs.

The succeeding sections of this report lay the foundation for the Committee's strategic vision for HIV prevention. Chapter 2 builds the case for a national surveillance system that identifies new HIV infections. Chapter 3 illustrates the value of allocating resources according to the cost and effectiveness of alternative programs, and it shows why evaluation is key to informing allocation decisions. Chapter 4 emphasizes the value still to be gained from closer integration of prevention into the clinical setting, and Chapter 5 points to the importance of filling the gap between research findings and effective action in the community. The promise of new technologies and the need for continued investment in research are the subject of Chapter 6. Finally, Chapter 7 tackles the underlying social conditions and attitudes that have hampered prevention efforts from the outset of the epidemic and continue to do so today.

Throughout its deliberations, the Committee has been motivated by the conviction that more can be done to prevent HIV infection. Doing better will require a new way of thinking about cost-effectiveness as a guiding principle for HIV prevention. It will require new leadership, accountability, and coordination; the Committee believes that, for HIV prevention efforts to have maximum impact, there must be a strong, clear leadership structure in the Department of Health and Human Services. Doing better will also require directing prevention efforts to those who are HIV-infected and those—women, youth, and racial and ethnic minorities—who are the new faces of the epidemic. It will require more effective translation of HIV prevention interventions that are successful in research settings into activities that are effective in communities. And it will require removing obstacles that impede the implementation of those interventions that we now know to be effective.

2

Tracking the Epidemic

Two decades after AIDS was first recognized in the United States, the epidemic continues to evolve in new directions. After a decade and a half of steady increase, AIDS incidence and AIDS deaths declined for the first time in 1996 (CDC, 1997), due to the development of newer and more effective antiretroviral therapies that slow disease progression and extend the lives of people with AIDS, and in part, to a combination of successful HIV prevention efforts. However, recent data suggest that the declines in AIDS incidence and deaths may be stabilizing (CDC, 2000a). At the same time, the number of people living with AIDS has steadily increased. Today, the number of people living with AIDS is at an all-time high (CDC, 2000b). The demographics of the epidemic also have changed considerably over time. While the proportion of AIDS cases among men who have sex with men has declined, the proportion of cases in women, youth, and racial and ethnic minorities has increased (CDC, 2000b). In addition, although the epidemic remains largely concentrated in urban areas, growth in AIDS cases in rural areas has been dramatic in recent years (CDC, 2000b) (see Appendix A for a more detailed discussion of the changing epidemic).

Much of what is known about the epidemic comes from the national AIDS case surveillance system. In this chapter, the Committee discusses the present system and its limitations, the rationale for implementing a surveillance approach to track the incidence of HIV, and the limitations of current HIV surveillance systems in measuring incidence. Further, the Committee recommends a new surveillance approach that can provide population-based estimates of HIV incidence.

NATIONAL AIDS SURVEILLANCE SYSTEM

Since the beginning of the epidemic, surveillance efforts have emphasized determining the number and characteristics of individuals diagnosed with AIDS. The current national AIDS case surveillance system, which was implemented prior to both the identification of HIV as the etiologic agent of AIDS and the development of an antibody test to determine HIV infection, was originally based on epidemiological investigations of an end-stage syndrome (Gostin et al., 1997). Each state requires that all patients diagnosed with AIDS be reported by name to the local, state, and/or territorial health departments. These reports are then forwarded (without names but with unique identifiers) to the Centers for Disease Control and Prevention (CDC), where a national surveillance database is created and analyzed. This surveillance system provides uniform data on trends and distribution of individuals diagnosed with AIDS. Standard records for each case include information on sex, race and ethnicity, state of residence (and metropolitan area, if relevant), mode of exposure to HIV, age at diagnosis, month of AIDS diagnosis, date reported, and other data. Although there are some reporting delays in the system, the data are relatively complete (more than 85 percent of AIDS cases) (Schwarcz et al., 1999; Buehler et al., 1992; Rosenblum et al., 1992) and statistical methods are available to adjust for both reporting delays and incompleteness (Green, 1998). Data from this surveillance system have been used as the basis for allocating federal resources for HIV treatment and care, and as the basis for planning local HIV prevention services (CDC, 1999a).

Until the era of potent antiretroviral therapies, AIDS case reporting, although imperfect, provided a relatively accurate picture of trends in HIV infection, especially relative HIV prevalence in groups defined by geography, race and ethnicity, and primary mode of infection. Estimates of HIV incidence and prevalence were made by statistical techniques, such as calculating backward from reported AIDS cases according to well-established patterns of disease progression (Brookmeyer and Gail, 1994). Recent developments in therapy for HIV and AIDS have at least temporally decoupled HIV infection and its progression to AIDS (Hammer et al., 1996; Collier et al., 1996). As a result, the timing of the progression from HIV infection to AIDS and from AIDS to death is increasingly difficult to predict, making HIV incidence and prevalence estimates based on AIDS cases much less accurate (CDC, 1999a). Consequently, AIDS case reporting is no longer adequate to monitor trends in HIV infection. The United States now faces the challenge of developing an effective HIV surveillance system that can predict where the epidemic is headed.

RATIONALE FOR A NATIONAL SYSTEM OF
HIV SURVEILLANCE

In considering how the current surveillance system might be optimally restructured, it is useful to examine the goals of surveillance and the types of data needed to achieve those goals. Public health officials, policy makers, researchers, and community groups use surveillance data to accomplish a variety of goals, including:

- tracking the course of the epidemic over time and place, in subpopulations, and by risk factors in order to assess its public health impact and to identify possible prevention strategies;
- evaluating access to and effectiveness of treatment and prevention efforts; and
- allocating resources for prevention, treatment, and care services, and for determining research priorities (Johri et al., 1998).

A variety of different types of data are needed to meet these goals. For example, data on HIV and AIDS incidence and prevalence, demographics, and risk factors are needed to track the course of the epidemic and to identify the populations needing treatment services. Incidence data are needed to judge the effectiveness of prevention programs and to set priorities for prevention programs (see Chapter 3). Optimally, an HIV surveillance system would also allow tabulation of sociodemographic and behavioral risk information on newly infected individuals which would offer a more precise picture of the HIV epidemic in the United States (see Text Box 2.1).

In its analysis and recommendations, the Committee makes the distinction between "surveillance" and "case finding." Surveillance is a *statistical* activity intended to provide for the "ongoing, systematic collection, analysis, interpretation, and dissemination of risk factor, exposure, and/or outcome-specific data for use in public health practice" (Thacker, 1994). Case finding, on the other hand, is intended to identify *individuals* who can benefit from early intervention in a disease process. Both surveillance and case finding rely on HIV testing, but for different purposes— surveillance to gather population-based data and case finding to identify infected individuals.

HIV CASE REPORTING

In response to concerns about the limitations of the current AIDS surveillance system in providing accurate information about trends in the HIV epidemic, the CDC recommends that all states and territories extend

---

TEXT BOX 2.1
Behavioral Surveillance

To help in improving the design and evaluation of prevention strategies, additional surveillance information is needed on behaviors that put people at risk for HIV. Currently, assessment of HIV risk behaviors is conducted on three levels. First, the CDC regularly conducts behavioral surveillance using such instruments as the Behavioral Risk Factor Surveillance System, the Youth Risk Behavior Surveillance System, and the National Survey for Family Growth (IOM, 1997). These surveys provide very general information about HIV testing and some sexual and drug use-related behaviors, but are very limited in the amount of data they provide regarding specific risk practices, particularly among high-risk subgroups, such as men who have sex with men and injection drug users. Behavioral surveys conducted among HIV-infected populations may provide information on practices that increase risk for viral transmission to sex and drug-using partners, but do not yield data on at-risk, uninfected persons. Behavioral assessments among high-risk populations fill this void, but often are constrained in their representativeness and generalizability due to sampling biases (e.g., as with convenience sampling).

Although each of these surveillance methods has limitations, together they might provide adequate information with which to better develop, implement, and evaluate prevention programs among populations at high risk of infection. The usefulness of data derived from these assessments, however, is often hampered by the lack of comparability between survey instruments and items that are intended to measure the same behavior (e.g., frequency of condom use). In order to provide some guidance in this matter, the CDC currently is developing a set of "core" items for use in HIV/STD behavioral surveillance surveys. This effort will be particularly useful in providing consistency for the measurement of sexual and drug use-related risk practices. Further, detailed information about the social contexts in which risk behaviors occur is sorely needed but rarely assessed. Assessments of such information should be integral components of behavioral assessments, as they serve to provide a better understanding of the dynamics of risk behavior and the social issues that need to be better addressed by prevention interventions. Therefore, the Committee endorses prior recommendations regarding the establishment of a national survey that can determine the prevalence and correlates of HIV risk-taking behavior (IOM, 1995).

---

their AIDS surveillance activities to include case reporting of HIV infection (CDC, 1999a). The CDC maintains that HIV case reporting will provide additional epidemiological data about HIV-infected populations to enhance prevention efforts, improve allocation of treatment resources, and assist in evaluating the impact of HIV prevention programs (CDC, 1999a). However, data from the HIV reporting system are incomplete in several important ways. In contrast to the AIDS case reporting system, which is relatively complete, the HIV reporting system collects data only from persons who choose to be tested and who do so at non-anonymous testing sites (i.e., where the HIV test result is linked with identifying information, including patient and provider names). Thus, HIV case reporting data exclude individuals who are infected but have not been tested, as well as those who use anonymous testing sites or home collection test kits (CDC, 1999a). Because of this selectivity, HIV case reporting by name is not representative of the larger population of infected persons. Further, because reported HIV cases could represent infections that are anywhere from a few weeks to a few years old, the data would reflect the time that individuals chose to be tested rather than when the individual became infected. As a result, HIV case reporting data provide only partial information about the number of existing HIV cases (HIV prevalence), rather than information about new HIV infections (HIV incidence) (Johri et al., 1998).

HIV case reporting can be implemented in one of two ways: through use of name reporting or through use of coded identifiers. As of June 1, 2000, a total of 35 states and the U.S. Virgin Islands had implemented HIV case surveillance using the same confidential name-based case reporting system used for AIDS cases. Two of these states (Connecticut and Oregon) conduct only pediatric HIV surveillance (CDC, 2000c). Name-based HIV case reporting has several potential benefits. First, name-based reporting can facilitate linkages between HIV case registries with those of other communicable diseases (e.g., syphilis and tuberculosis) at the state and local level. This cross-referencing can be used by public health officials to obtain a more comprehensive picture of their local epidemic and effectively target local level prevention and care services (K. Toomey, personal communication). Name-based reporting has also been suggested as a case-finding method by which HIV-infected individuals could be linked to treatment services (Colfax and Bindman, 1998). However, reporting HIV cases to state health departments does not automatically ensure that HIV-infected persons will receive beneficial linkages to care.[1] In a recent study, Osmond and colleagues (1999) found that contact with a health department after testing HIV-infected was not associated with receipt of timelier care. Finally, HIV name-based reporting may enhance partner notification programs that are used to identify individuals at high risk of infection (Colfax and Bindman, 1998).[2]

One of the major concerns with name-based reporting is the potential for breaches of confidentiality. For example, groups that were both heavily affected by HIV/AIDS and already stigmatized by society (e.g., gay men

---

[1]For instance, although the potential benefit exists, states historically have not used their AIDS registries to ensure access to care (Johri et al., 1998).

[2]Name-based reporting is not necessary for partner notification, however, because people can identify their partners without identifying themselves (Colfax and Bindman, 1998).

and injection drug users) initially felt that compiling a list of the names of HIV-infected persons would compound the stigma they were already experiencing. There also were concerns that such a list could be used for discriminatory purposes should it become publicly available (Gostin et al., 1997). However, there have been very few reported incidents of intentional misuse of this information (Colfax and Bindman, 1998). In addition, there is substantial concern that name-based reporting may deter individuals at risk of infection from being tested, thus delaying their access to counseling or treatment services (Colfax and Bindman, 1998; Woods et al., 1999). Some studies have suggested that name-based reporting policies might deter or postpone some high-risk individuals from seeking testing (CDC, 1998; Hecht et al., 1997, 2000). For these reasons, the CDC supports adherence to strict confidentiality protections of testing and surveillance data and the availability of anonymous testing options (CDC, 1999a).

Concerns that stigma, discrimination, and breaches in confidentiality might deter some individuals from being tested have led some states such as Maryland and Massachusetts to implement a coded system of HIV case reporting based on "unique identifiers" (CDC, 1999a; Solomon et al., 1999). This system is similar to HIV name-based case reporting, except a code number is created and reported rather than the individual's name. Each code number is based on information specific to the individual (e.g., Social Security number). If all elements of the code are complete and accurate, the code number is unique enough to avoid duplicate records (Solomon et al., 1999), while still allowing for follow-up to obtain additional information.

While the unique identifier case reporting system does address concerns about confidentiality, the data obtained from this type of surveillance have the same statistical drawbacks as name-based reporting with regard to timeliness and test site selection bias. Although both systems provide data that are, in a sense, more timely than AIDS case reporting for estimating HIV incidence, they still provide an incomplete and inaccurate picture of the HIV epidemic.

POPULATION-BASED HIV INCIDENCE ESTIMATION

In order to meet the goal of providing accurate HIV incidence information, a new surveillance approach is needed. With this in mind, the Committee proposes the use of sentinel surveillance, a method that would obtain incidence data from targeted samples of "sentinel" populations using advanced testing technology, in combination with statistical modeling to extrapolate these incidence data to larger subsets of the population or the population as a whole (Johri et al., 1998).

Current estimates of HIV/AIDS prevalence and incidence are based in part on a "family of surveys" in a variety of populations: screening results of blood samples derived from programs testing special populations (e.g., blood donors and applicants to the military and Job Corps) and testing of anonymous blood specimens from smaller studies (e.g., at sexually transmitted disease clinics, drug treatment centers, and adolescent medical clinics) (Pappaioanou et al., 1990). These surveys, however, draw from non-representative convenience samples rather than from probability samples.[3] As a result, many sources of potential bias exist. Changes in measurement techniques also introduce bias. For example, the group tested may not be representative of the population, or the populations being tested may not be stable over time.

Restructuring the family of HIV surveys to permit better statistical estimates would optimize knowledge of HIV incidence. Indeed, the National Research Council (NRC) has recommended that the CDC family of surveys be reformulated as two-stage probability samples (NRC, 1989). First, a random sample of nationwide drug treatment centers, sentinel hospitals and primary care facilities, clinics devoted to sexually transmitted diseases and tuberculosis, and clinics serving women of reproductive age would be chosen. For reasons of statistical efficiency, settings that are likely to serve a large number of HIV-infected persons, such as drug treatment centers, should be more intensively sampled. However, in order to get nationally and locally representative estimates, sampling should not be limited to such sites. Second, random samples of blood from clients of these facilities would be chosen and tested anonymously for HIV. Thus, the survey sites must be ones in which blood is normally drawn for routine testing. The clustered nature of the final sample must be taken into account in determining the appropriate sizes of the first and second size samples. Additionally, in order to extrapolate to a broader population of individuals who visit these sites, questions would be added to nationally representative surveys, such as the National Health Interview Survey, about whether individuals had visited the kind of facilities targeted by the family of HIV serosurveys. With these results, accurate statistical estimates can be made of the prevalence of HIV in demographically defined groups. Reinstating some representative subset of the Survey of Childbearing Women, which was based on anonymous HIV testing of newborn

---

[3]Convenience samples draw from a population that is readily accessible, but that may not be representative of the population of interest. In contrast, in probability samples, all members of the population of interest have a known probability of being in the sample, allowing researchers to develop population-based estimates (Wilcox and Marks, 1994).

children and which was discontinued by the CDC in 1994, also would be an important part of this effort.

Further, the recommended serosurveillance effort should also incorporate the use of recent advances in HIV testing, such as the detuned assay (Janssen et al., 1998). The detuned assay is an advanced testing technique that determines whether an individual has been infected with HIV within approximately the past four to six months[4] (Janssen et al., 1998, CDC, 1999b). Combined with probability sampling approaches (Kaplan and Brookmeyer, 1999) that would improve estimates of HIV prevalence, the use of detuned assays could yield more accurate national estimates of HIV incidence. It should be noted that because blood samples are tested anonymously, sentinel serosurveillance methodologies are not suitable for facilitating linkages to care.

Surveillance systems can be evaluated in terms of a number of characteristics, including simplicity, flexibility, acceptability, sensitivity (the ability to include existing cases), positive predictive value (the likelihood that included cases do in fact have the intended disease or condition), representativeness (the ability to describe the occurrence of a health event over time and its distribution in the population by place and personal characteristics), and timeliness (Buehler, 1998). Table 2.1 compares the alternative approaches using three of these criteria (timeliness, representativeness, acceptability).

From this analysis, the Committee concludes that a new surveillance system focused on HIV incidence is needed in order to more effectively guide HIV prevention planning, resource allocation, and evaluation decisions at the national, state, and local levels. To the extent possible, the system would provide estimates at the state and local level and for the population groups at highest risk for HIV infection. We believe that a system of population-based HIV incidence estimation will provide the most accurate and timely data for these objectives. Too often, surveillance data are haphazardly collected as incidental by-products of clinical or social services to selected patients rather than as part of a coordinated strategy. To reflect the importance of HIV/AIDS to our society and to do a better job of allocating scarce resources for HIV prevention (see Chapter 3) a more effective surveillance system is needed. Therefore, the Committee recommends that:

---

[4]Specifically, two different enzyme immunoassay tests for HIV antibodies would be performed on each individual. The first test is a standard, highly sensitive version, while the second test is a less sensitive "detuned" version. Individuals who test positive on the first test but negative on the second of this "sensitive assay, less sensitive assay" testing series would be identified as recently infected (Janssen et al., 1998).

TABLE 2.1 Comparison of HIV Surveillance Approaches

Surveillance Approach	Timeliness (re: HIV infection)	Representativeness	Acceptability
HIV case reporting by name	Dependent on HIV testing behaviors	Bisiased based on who tested; includes only those tested confidentially	Possibility of stigma, discrimination, and deterrence from testing
HIV case reporting by unique identifier (ID)	Dependent on HIV testing behaviors	Less test avoidance to avoid reporting to authorities	Reduced possibility of stigma, discrimination, and deterrence from testing
Population-based incidence estimation	Can estimate new infections	Relatively unbiased	Minimal risk of stigma and discrimination because testing is blinded

NOTE: Because the Committee is concerned with identifying an optimal surveillance method, the Committee does not consider in this analysis whether these approaches fulfill case-finding objectives, such as linking individuals to care or conducting partner notification.

The Centers for Disease Control and Prevention create a surveillance system that can provide national population-based estimates of HIV incidence. The recommended surveillance system would estimate new HIV infections using blinded serosurveys of well-characterized sentinel populations (e.g., drug users in treatment, people attending sexually transmitted disease clinics and tuberculosis clinics, clinics serving women of reproductive age), surveys that characterize the populations served by those sites, and advanced testing technologies that are able to identify recent HIV infections.

The Committee is aware that previous attempts to do HIV surveillance have been controversial (Bayer, 1997), particularly before effective therapies became available. In the 1980s, some groups perceived the "public health" responses to AIDS as being aimed at identifying HIV carriers and protecting the blood supply, without any regard for the rights or protection of those infected. In the 1990s, legislation to mandate HIV testing of newborn children without the consent of their mothers (whose HIV antibodies were actually being tested) added to the distrust of public health officials that was already felt by some groups (IOM, 1999). Thus, in many quarters, HIV case reporting seemed to offer little to HIV-infected people.

Now that effective therapies are available and individuals have a variety of opportunities for confidential HIV testing, there are strong reasons for people to be tested if for no other reason than to protect their own health. However knowing one's serostatus is only helpful if it results in obtaining medical care and treatment for HIV infection. The Committee's proposal for HIV surveillance based on anonymous test results at sentinel sites separates surveillance (a statistical activity) from case finding, and it has the potential to both provide better estimates of HIV incidence and avoid the controversies of case reporting. HIV case finding, used for linking infected persons to care, partner notification, or contact tracing, is a separate prevention activity and should be judged in reference to other uses of prevention funds (see Chapter 3).

REFERENCES

Bayer R. 1997. Science, politics, and AIDS prevention policy. *Journal of Acquired Immune Deficiency Syndrome and Human Retrovirology* 14 (Suppl 2):S22–S29.

Brookmeyer R and Gail MH. 1994. *AIDS Epidemiology: A Quantitative Approach.* New York: Oxford University Press.

Buehler JW. 1998. Surveillance. In Rothman KJ and Greenland S, (Eds.), *Modern Epidemiology,* 2nd ed. Philadelphia: Lippincott Williams and Williams.

Buehler JW, Berkelman RL, Stehr-Green JK. 1992. The completeness of AIDS surveillance. *Journal of Acquired Immune Deficiency Syndrome* 5(3):257–264.

Centers for Disease Control and Prevention (CDC). 2000a. U.S. AIDS Cases, Deaths, and HIV Infections Appear Stable. AMA Press Briefing, July 8.

Centers for Disease Control and Prevention (CDC). 2000b. HIV/AIDS Surveillance Report, 1999 11(2). Atlanta: CDC.

Centers for Disease Control and Prevention (CDC). 2000c. Current Status of HIV Infection Reporting— May 2000. Atlanta: CDC.

Centers for Disease Control and Prevention (CDC). 1999a. Guidelines for national human immunodeficiency virus case surveillance, including monitoring for human immunodeficiency virus infection and acquired immunodeficiency syndrome. *Morbidity and Mortality Weekly Report* 48(RR-13):1–31.

Centers for Disease Control and Prevention (CDC). 1999b. New HIV Test Provides Unprecedented Look at Level of New Infections in High-Risk Groups. Press Briefing. 1999 National Prevention Conference. August 29 – September 1. Atlanta, GA.

Centers for Disease Control and Prevention (CDC). 1998. HIV testing among populations at risk for HIV infection—nine states. *Morbidity and Mortality Weekly Report* 47:1086–1091.

Centers for Disease Control and Prevention (CDC). 1997. Update: Trends in AIDS incidence—United States, 1996. *Morbidity and Mortality Weekly Report* 46:861–867.

Colfax GN and Bindman AB. 1998. Health benefits and risks of reporting HIV-infected individuals by name. *American Journal of Public Health* 88(6):876–879.

Collier AC, Coombs RW, Schoenfeld DA, Bassett RL, Timpone J, Baruch A, Jones M, Facey K, Whitacre C, McAuliffe VJ, Friedman HM, Merigan TC, Reichman RC, Hooper C, Corey L. 1996. Treatment of human immunodeficiency virus infection with saquinavir, zidovudine, and zalcitabine. AIDS Clinical Trials Group. *New England Journal of Medicine* 334(16):1011–1017.

Gostin LO, Ward JW, Baker AC. 1997. National HIV case reporting for the United States. A defining moment in the history of the epidemic. *New England Journal of Medicine* 337(16):1162–1167.

Green TA. 1998. Using surveillance data to monitor trends in the AIDS epidemic. *Statistics in Medicine* (2):143–154.

Hammer SM, Katzenstein DA, Hughes MD, Gundacker H, Schooley RT, Haubrich RH, Henry WK, Lederman MM, Phair JP, Niu M, Hirsch MS, Merigan TC. 1996. A trial comparing nucleoside monotherapy with combination therapy in HIV-infected adults with CD4 cell counts from 200 to 500 per cubic millimeter. AIDS Clinical Trials Group Study 175 Study Team. *New England Journal of Medicine* 335(15):1081–1090.

Hecht FM, Chesney MA, Lehman JS, Osmond D, Vranizan K, Colman S, Keane D, Reingold A, Bindman AB. 2000. Does HIV reporting by name deter testing? MESH Study Group. *AIDS* 14(12):1801–1808.

Hecht FM, Coleman S, Lehman JS, Vranizan K, Keane D, Bindman AB, Chesney M, and the MESH Study Group, San Francisco General Hospital, UCSF, San Francisco, CA, and CDC, Atlanta, GA. 1997. Named reporting of HIV: Attitudes and knowledge of those at risk (Abstract). *Journal of General Internal Medicine* 12(Suppl 1):108.

Institute of Medicine. 1999. *Reducing the Odds: Preventing Perinatal Transmission of HIV in the United States.* Stoto MA, Almario DA, and McCormick MC (Eds.). Washington, DC: National Academy Press.

Institute of Medicine. 1997. *The Hidden Epidemic: Confronting Sexually Transmitted Diseases.* Eng T and Butler W (Eds.). Washington, DC: National Academy Press.

Institute of Medicine. 1995. *AIDS and Behavior: An Integrated Approach.* Auerbach J, Wypijewska C, and Brodie K (Eds.). Washington, DC: National Academy Press.

Janssen RS, Satten GA, Stramer SL, Rawal BD, O'Brien TR, Weiblen BJ, Hecht FM, Jack N, Cleghorn FR, Kahn JO, Chesney MA, Busch MP. 1998. New testing strategy to detect early HIV-1 infection for use in incidence estimates and for clinical and prevention purposes. *Journal of the American Medical Association* 280(1):42–48.

Johri M, Kaplan EH, Levi J, Novick A. 1998. New approaches to HIV surveillance: Means and ends. A Summary Report of the Law, Policy, and Ethics Conference on HIV Surveillance, May 21–22, 1998. Yale University Center for Interdisciplinary Research on AIDS.

Kaplan EH and Brookmeyer R. 1999. Snapshot estimators of recent HIV incidence rates. *Operations Research* 47(1):29–37.

National Research Council. 1989. *AIDS: Sexual Behavior and Intravenous Drug Use.* Turner CF, Miller HG, and Moses LE (Eds.). Washington, DC: National Academy Press.

Osmond DH, Bindman AB, Vranizan K, Lehman JS, Hecht FM, Keane D, Reingold A. 1999. Name-based surveillance and public health interventions for persons with HIV infection. Multistate Evaluation of Surveillance for HIV Study Group. *Annals of Internal Medicine* 131(10):775–779.

Pappaioanou M, Dondero TJ Jr, Petersen LR, Onorato IM, Sanchez CD, Curran JW. 1990. The family of HIV seroprevalence surveys: Objectives, methods, and uses of sentinel surveillance for HIV in the United States. *Public Health Reports* 105(2):113–119.

Rosenblum L, Buehler JW, Morgan MW, Costa S, Hidalgo J, Holmes R, Lieb L, Shields A, Whyte BM. 1992. The completeness of AIDS case reporting, 1988: A multisite collaborative surveillance project. *American Journal of Public Health* 82(11):1495–1499.

Schwarcz SK, Hsu LC, Parisi MK, Katz MH. 1999. The impact of the 1993 AIDS case definition on the completeness and timeliness of AIDS surveillance. *AIDS* 13(9):1109–1114.

Solomon L, Flynn C, Caldeira E, Wasserman MP, Benjamin G. 1999. Evaluation of a statewide non-name-based HIV surveillance system. *Journal of Acquired Immunodeficiency Syndromes* 22:272–279.

Thacker SB. 1994. Historical Development. In Teutsch SM and Churchill RE. (Eds.), *Principles and Practice of Public Health Surveillance*. New York: Oxford University Press.

Toomey K. Georgia Department of Human Resources, Personal Communication, June 16, 2000.

Wilcox LS and Marks JS. 1994. Overview. *From Data to Action: CDC's Public Health Surveillance for Women, Infants and Children*. Atlanta: CDC.

Woods WJ, Dilley JW, Lihatsh T, Sabatino J, Adler B, Rinaldi J. 1997. Name-based reporting of HIV-positive test results as a deterrent to testing. *American Journal of Public Health* 89(7):1097–1100.

3

Allocating Resources

The Committee was charged, in part, with recommending a vision-ary framework for effective HIV prevention in the United States over the next 5 years. The Committee began by reviewing the HIV prevention literature. This review not only illustrated the wide variety of available social, behavioral, and technological interventions, but also high-lighted the dramatic successes that have been accomplished through pre-vention (see Appendix B for more detail). The Committee also examined the sources and levels of federal funding for HIV prevention. We focused in particular on the Centers for Disease Control and Prevention (CDC), which plays a leading role in HIV prevention, although numerous other federal, state, and local government, and private agencies contribute sub-stantially to these efforts (see Appendix C for a description of federal HIV prevention efforts). Further, the Committee examined the implicit strate-gies that appear to currently drive the investment of HIV prevention dollars, and we compared the results of those investments to the results that might have been achieved if those same resources had been allocated based on the new goal that we propose in this report, that is, preventing as many new HIV infections as possible.

The Committee's analysis was challenging for numerous reasons, in-cluding the difficulty of determining exactly how current federal HIV funds are being spent, the absence of reliable data on HIV infection rates, and the limited data on the effectiveness and costs of many prevention interventions.[1] Nevertheless, the Committee believes that decisions regarding the allocation of public HIV prevention funds represent the single most important set of HIV prevention decisions made. Further, the Committee's analysis indicates that a clear, consistently applied strategy of investing prevention funds in interventions that achieve the greatest potential reduction in new HIV infections could increase significantly the number of HIV infections prevented, even within current funding levels. Under this strategy, prevention funds would be allocated to the groups at highest risk and to the interventions that produce the biggest payoff for each dollar invested.

Today, very few policy makers or program administrators recognize either the enormous variation that exists in the cost-effectiveness of different types of programs or the importance of this variation in the overall impact of HIV prevention programs on the epidemic. Economic evaluation has emerged in recent years as an important tool for assisting in health policy decisions, and is increasingly being applied in the HIV prevention field (Holtgrave, 1998). Several major efforts have now examined the role of economic evaluation in public health policy decisions and have addressed methodological issues in conducting these evaluations (Phillips et al., 1998). For instance, the CDC has developed a practical guide to economic evaluation and decision analysis in public health policy decisions (Teutsch and Haddix, 1994; Haddix et al., 1996). The Panel on Cost-Effectiveness in Health and Medicine, convened by the U.S. Public Health Service in 1993, also has provided suggestions for improving the quality and comparability of cost-effectiveness analyses in health care decisions (Gold et al., 1996). In addition, collaborators from the CDC, local governments, academia, industry, and the Task Force on Community Preventive Services have established guidelines for systematic reviews of economic evaluations in community prevention (Carande-Kulis et al., 2000) and are currently examining the cost-effectiveness of HIV prevention interventions.

Still, it is unrealistic to expect that all federal prevention funds will be redirected to interventions that are shown to be the most cost-effective in

---

[1]Throughout this chapter, the Committee uses the terms "HIV prevention programs," "HIV prevention interventions," or "HIV prevention activities" to refer to publicly sponsored actions intended to prevent new HIV infections. Sometimes the Committee discusses specific interventions (such as needle exchange or HIV counseling and testing), while at other times, the Committee discusses a portfolio of activities (such as interventions addressing the needs of injection drug users or men who have sex with men). On occasion, the Committee alludes to federal agency programmatic categories (such as health education and risk reduction efforts sponsored by the CDC). The specific meaning of terms like program, intervention, or activity in any instance will be clear from the context.

preventing new HIV infections, as resource allocation decisions are made in a highly charged environment, subject to numerous competing influences, including politics, advocacy, scientific evidence, personal values, and community norms (Holtgrave, 1998). However, a reassessment of current program investments, along with a strong commitment to direct all future increases in funding according to the principle of preventing the largest number of new infections, will yield meaningful results. The Committee recognizes the technical, social, and political barriers to immediate acceptance of this approach, but believes that the evidence argues strongly for a prevention strategy based on this principle.

In this chapter, the Committee argues the case for a data-driven strategy in support of programs that 1) demonstrate success in preventing new HIV infections and 2) do so on a cost-effective basis. Models that estimate the impact of adopting this strategy suggest that it will produce significant reductions in rates of new infections.

CURRENT ALLOCATION OF FEDERAL
HIV PREVENTION FUNDS

Federal spending on HIV/AIDS is enormously complex and divided among numerous departments and agencies across the federal government. Within the Department of Health and Human Services alone, multiple agencies, including the CDC, the National Institutes of Health (NIH), the Substance Abuse and Mental Health Services Administration (SAMHSA), and the Health Resources Services Administration (HRSA), share responsibility for HIV prevention, research, and treatment efforts. State and localities also play a significant role in deciding how federal HIV prevention funds are spent. For instance, the CDC distributes a significant portion ($258 million in fiscal year 1999) of its total HIV prevention budget ($678 million in fiscal year 1999) through cooperative agreements with 65 state and local health departments (CDC, 1999). Community Planning Groups, comprised of representatives from groups of people at risk for HIV infection and of providers of HIV prevention services, advise these state and local health departments in setting their priorities and in making programmatic and resource allocation decisions (Valdiserri et al., 1995; Kaplan, 1998; Kaplan and Pollack, 1998). Similarly, SAMHSA distributes Substance Abuse Prevention and Treatment (SAPT) block grant funds to states, which decide how these funds and SAPT HIV set-aside funds[2] will be used at the state and local level. Decisions regard-

---

[2]Qualifying states, with an AIDS case rate of 10 per 100,000 population, are required to set aside between two and five percent of their SAPT block grant funds for HIV early intervention services (SAMHSA, 2000a).

ing the majority of Ryan White CARE Act funds, administered by HRSA, are also made at the state and local level (HRSA, 2000).[3]

Thus, there is no explicit strategy that currently guides the overall investment of federal HIV prevention funds. In some cases, individual agencies provide general criteria for prioritizing the use of federal funds. For example, the CDC directs Community Planning Groups to prioritize funds on the basis of several factors, including documented need, scientific evidence (including cost-effectiveness), consumer values and preferences, and local circumstances (CDC, 1993; Valdiserri et al., 1995). Other resource allocation decisions are subject to congressional mandates or earmarks. In many other cases, however, the criteria used to make decisions are less obvious. For instance, while Congress provides direction on the types of activities that the SAPT block grant and HIV set-aside funds can support, states have considerable discretion in how these funds are allocated. Currently, there is little information about the criteria that states use in their decisions, the types of activities that the SAPT block grant and HIV set-aside funds support, and the effectiveness or quality of programs that are funded (GAO, 2000).

Many prevention policy and funding decisions appear to be made with the tacit goal of avoiding political interference. For example, a 1994 external review suggested that CDC's HIV prevention efforts had been limited and distorted by political pressures from the Reagan and Bush Administrations (Bayer, 1997). Fear of political reprise has been cited by some observers as a major factor in the Clinton Administration's decision not to rescind the ban on federal funding of needle exchange programs, despite clear scientific evidence as to the value of such programs (Stolberg, 1998). Political factors also contributed to the CDC's decision to suspend the Survey of Childbearing Women, which involved anonymous HIV testing of infants for surveillance purposes. This survey was halted just as Congress was pushing legislation to unblind the test results, a measure which would reveal the mother's HIV status, but not necessarily the infant's HIV status (Burr, 1997; IOM, 1999).

Indeed, the distribution of federal funds can best be described as an amalgam of administrative and legislative decisions that have been shaped in response to available data, constituency pressures, congressional mandates and earmarks, personal values, and the professional judgment of program managers. Further, the strategy that results from these cumulative decisions can best be described as "proportionality." For the most part, federal HIV prevention funds—and CDC funds in particular—

---

[3]The CARE Act primarily funds HIV treatment services, but also funds some prevention services.

are broadly allocated to maintain proportionality to reported AIDS cases. Thus, proportionality is the implicit strategy for allocation of federal funds. This point is illustrated by Figures 3.1–3.4. Figures 3.1 and 3.2 show how, over time, funds distributed to programs in two different CDC program categories providing services to different racial/ethnic groups approached the proportion of AIDS cases in these groups. Figures 3.3 and 3.4 show that community-planning funds distributed by the CDC to states to support HIV prevention were roughly proportional to the number of new AIDS cases reported by the states.

As a prevention strategy, proportionality has one important advantage. It begins with an objective criterion of need: observed AIDS cases. While proportionality may be useful for allocating funds for AIDS treatment, it has serious limitations, including the fact that it is an inadequate marker of need for prevention services. Further, proportionality rewards the reporting of AIDS cases rather than the prevention of new infections. This has the potential for creating two serious inefficiencies. First, proportionality reflects where the epidemic has been, rather than where it is going. Second, it rewards states and localities that use their resources ineffectively—and, as a result, have unnecessarily higher caseloads. The Committee believes that the adoption of a more sophisticated strategy

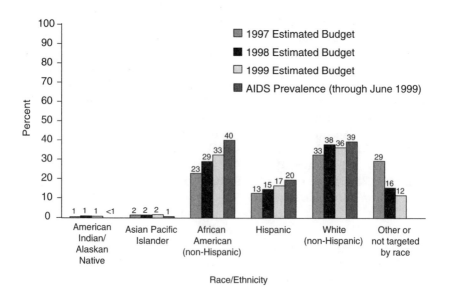

FIGURE 3.1 Counseling, testing, referral, and partner notification: FY 1997 to FY 1999 budget projections compared with AIDS prevalence by race/ethnicity. NOTE: AIDS not reported for other or not targeted by race/ethnicity. SOURCE: CDC.

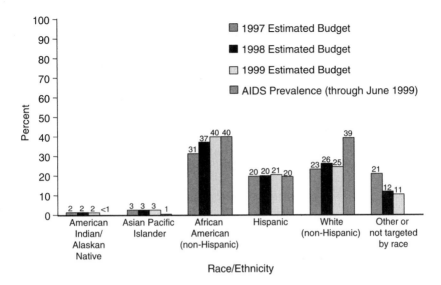

FIGURE 3.2 Health education and risk reduction: FY 1997 to FY 1999 budget projections compared with AIDS prevalence by race/ethnicity. NOTE: AIDS not reported for other or not targeted by race/ethnicity. SOURCE: CDC.

will yield larger returns. As an alternative to proportionality, the Committee recommends that prevention funds be allocated to reach populations at highest risk and to support programs that are cost-effective. Both aims are necessary to support a strategy of preventing the greatest number of new infections within budget constraints.

The Committee believes that it is now possible to start basing resource allocation decisions on cost-effectiveness principles. Cost-effectiveness is as much a way of thinking as a formal, quantitative technique for conducting policy analysis (Holtgrave, 1998). Since 1994, the CDC has endorsed the use of cost-effectiveness data as one component of its resource allocation decisions (Valdiserri et al., 1995). Even with imperfect information, adopting this framework of thinking about HIV prevention investment can set the stage for substantial improvements. While employing a framework of cost-effectiveness cannot dissolve the constraints on HIV prevention imposed by laws or the pressures of Congress, nor can it alleviate the social barriers (e.g., stigma, poverty, racism) that continue to fuel the epidemic and shape prevention policy (see Chapter 7), refocusing allocation decisions on the basis of cost-effectiveness can help elevate the discussion beyond these factors. The Committee believes that federal and state agencies, using the analytic findings to date, could make better decisions regarding their investments. Adopting a cost-effectiveness

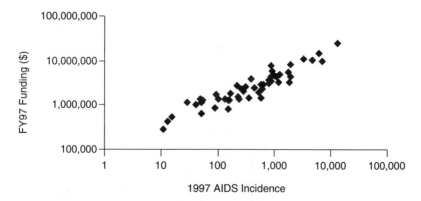

FIGURE 3.3 CDC-Allocated HIV prevention funds versus AIDS incidence by state.

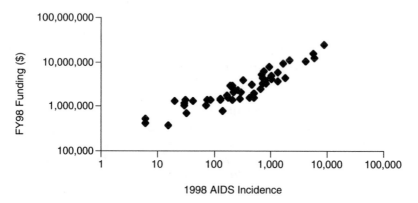

FIGURE 3.4 CDC-Allocated HIV prevention funds versus AIDS incidence by state.

framework will also point decision makers to areas where data are lacking and further research is warranted. In the absence of this framework, policy makers will continue to use the same decision rules that previously have failed in the past to maximize the number of HIV infections averted.

ASSESSING THE COST-EFFECTIVENESS OF
HIV PREVENTION INTERVENTIONS

The cost-effectiveness of an intervention is a product of two factors: the cost of the intervention and the number of new infections prevented. The number of infections prevented by any particular intervention depends on the baseline rate of new infections in the population that would occur in the absence of the intervention, and the fraction of those infections that the intervention can avert. Estimating the baseline rate of new infections (aggregate HIV incidence) is a problem of HIV epidemiology, while estimating program effectiveness is the fundamental challenge of program evaluation (Kaplan, 1998).

Researchers are working in both of these areas, but rarely have they converged to combine estimates for both factors.[4] The Committee has attempted to combine these two areas to illustrate the value of an investment-based approach to allocation of prevention funds. Policy makers are not accustomed to making allocation decisions on the basis of cost-effectiveness. First, data have not been available to make decisions on that basis. Further, other values have dominated policy decisions about which interventions to support. The three examples below illustrate this point.

Protecting the Blood Supply

All blood donations in the United States have been screened for HIV since the deployment of the HIV antibody test in 1985, and this screening has reduced sharply the number of transfusion-related AIDS cases. However, screening is not 100 percent effective. There is a "window period" between the time of infection and the time when HIV antibodies can be detected by the screening test, and blood donated during this period may carry the AIDS virus. The window period for the recombinant HIV-1/2 combination enzyme-linked immunoassay (EIA) test is estimated at 22 days (Petersen et al., 1994; Busch et al., 1995; GAO, 1998). The p24 antigen assay, used since 1996, has reduced the window to about 16 days (Busch et al., 1995; AuBuchon et al., 1997; GAO, 1998). This six-day reduction lowered the number of infectious donations that entered the blood supply by about 27 percent. The absolute number of infections prevented, however, has been modest because the blood supply already was very safe. An estimated eight additional transfusion-related cases of HIV were pre-

---

[4] A variety of procedures have been developed for estimating HIV incidence, including epidemiological cohort studies and back-calculation from AIDS cases (Brookmeyer and Gail, 1994). Approaches developed more recently, such as the detuned assay (Janssen et al., 1998) and snapshot estimators (Kaplan and Brookmeyer, 1999), hold promise for the spot estimation of HIV incidence among subpopulations in specific settings. The use of such techniques in conjunction with the new surveillance approach recommended by the Committee could enable reasonably accurate estimates of HIV incidence by state and area. For examples of attempts to estimate the number of HIV infections averted by interventions, see Holtgrave (1998) and Kaplan (1995).

vented, producing a cost-effectiveness ratio of *$7.5 million per HIV infection prevented*, compared to HIV antibody screening alone. Through extensive clinical trials, the Food and Drug Administration (FDA) has encouraged the development and use of a new, extremely sensitive Nucleic Acid Amplification Technology (NAT) test. This technology is designed to provide additional protection by further reducing the window period. Each additional HIV infection prevented with this new test will likely come at an even higher cost.

Preventing Perinatal Transmission of HIV

Approximately 6,000 to 7,000 HIV-infected women in the United States become pregnant each year (IOM, 1999). In the absence of treatment, between 25 percent and 30 percent of the babies born to these women will also be HIV-infected. However, the antiretroviral drug zidovudine (ZDV) has been proven effective in reducing the transmission probability to between 2 and 5 percent (IOM, 1999). The widespread use of ZDV, nevirapine, and other antiretroviral medications[5] in the United States has prevented approximately 1,560 cases of perinatal HIV transmission annually. Combining the $5,700 cost of treatment for HIV-infected mothers with the HIV screening costs for all pregnant women in the United States results in a total estimated cost of $51 million, and a cost-effectiveness estimate of roughly *$32,700 per HIV infection prevented*.

Implementing Needle Exchange Programs

Injection drug users (IDUs) may account for an estimated 50 percent of new HIV infections (Holmberg, 1996), making them an obvious priority group for HIV prevention. Needle exchange programs that enable IDUs to trade used needles and syringes for clean equipment have proven valuable and cost-effective in HIV prevention. Many published evaluations of needle exchange programs, including separate reviews by the National Research Council, the CDC, and the U.S. General Accounting Office, have concluded that such programs reduce the spread of HIV without increasing the incidence of drug abuse in the community (GAO, 1993; NRC, 1995). Depending on the specific program model employed,

---

[5]The most recent Public Health Service Task Force recommendations for the use of antiretroviral drugs in HIV-infected pregnant women call for the use of combination antiretroviral drug therapy to maximally suppress the virus and prevent perinatal transmission (CDC, 2000).

the cost-effectiveness of needle exchange is estimated to range from *$3,000 to $50,000 per HIV infection prevented* (Kaplan, 1995; Kahn, 1998), figures that are competitive with the cost-effectiveness of zidovudine for preventing perinatal transmission. However, needle exchange programs are not widely employed due to syringe prescription laws in some states and the prohibition against using federal funds to support such programs (See Chapter 7 for a discussion of needle exchange policies).

These examples illustrate how the federal government has promoted certain interventions and avoided others. In certain areas, large sums of money have been spent to prevent a small incremental number of infections; in other areas, federal policy prohibits federal sponsorship of certain interventions that have been proven effective in preventing a substantially larger number of infections. Together, these decisions imply a very wide range of implicit valuations regarding the monetary value of preventing an HIV infection. These decisions suggest, for example, that society implicitly values preventing a transfusion-related infection 150 times more ($7.5 million per infection averted) than preventing a drug-related infection through needle exchange ($50,000 per infection averted). While some variation in these values is to be reasonably expected,[6] it is difficult to reconcile a difference of such magnitude.

USING EPIDEMIC IMPACT AS A MEASURE OF SUCCESS

In the examples above, data exist to make reasonably accurate estimates of both the impact of the intervention on new HIV infections, or the "epidemic impact," and the cost of each new infection averted. Such clear evidence rarely is available. The Committee reviewed numerous studies evaluating HIV prevention interventions. Many of the studies conclude that "prevention works"—and, in the immediate frame of reference of the intervention, they may be correct. The great majority of such studies present comparisons of self-reported HIV risk behaviors among those participating in an HIV prevention intervention before and after the intervention was launched, and often in comparison with individuals who did

---

[6]The Committee acknowledges that some people may place a higher value on preventing an infection through the blood supply than through needle exchange, for several reasons. Factors that could contribute to this higher valuation might include perceptions about lack of control over transfusion-related infections, the additional benefits of preventing hepatitis and other blood-borne illnesses through transfusion, or maintaining public confidence in the blood supply. Without attempting to pin down a precise valuation for preventing infections through transfusion versus needle sharing, however, the Committee questions whether the implicit difference in values is reasonable.

not receive the intervention. Typically, interventions are deemed successful if there are statistically significant changes in self-reported behaviors
in the appropriate direction. For example, in an intervention designed to
get men to use condoms during sex, if the average number of times men
use condoms increases beyond what chance fluctuations would predict,
then the intervention is viewed as a success. Likewise, if injection drug
users participating in an intervention report that they are sharing needles
less often, then this is taken as evidence that "prevention works."

The intent here is not to review the difficulties inherent in the study of
HIV risk behaviors (see NRC, 1991, for such a review). Rather, the Committee wishes to point out that, even if the reported social and behavioral
data in HIV prevention studies are completely accurate, it remains difficult to decide what the results really mean in terms of HIV prevention.
The basic question is: how many HIV infections can be averted through
the deployment of alternative prevention interventions?

Consider the example of a prevention intervention that induces men
to increase from 10 percent to 20 percent the rate at which they use
condoms during receptive anal intercourse—a doubling of condom use.
Assuming that the frequency with which these men practice such intercourse remains unchanged, the intervention would have doubled the
number of protected acts of anal intercourse. This seems like strong evidence in favor of the intervention. However, from the standpoint of averting HIV infections, 90 percent of all acts of anal intercourse were unprotected before the intervention while, following the intervention, 80 percent
of all such acts were unprotected. Basic principles of epidemiology suggest that the incidence of new HIV infections among receptive partners
will be proportional to both HIV prevalence among insertive partners
and the rate of unprotected anal intercourse (Anderson and May, 1991;
Kahn, 1996). Since HIV prevalence would not change over a short time
period, the relative reduction in HIV incidence is on the order of the
relative reduction in the rate of unprotected anal intercourse, which equals
11 percent. Thus, a doubling of condom use in this example would lead
only to an 11 percent reduction in HIV incidence.

This illustrates the point that, in considering the effectiveness of HIV
prevention interventions for purposes of allocating funds, it is important
to assess the potential benefits of prevention in terms of epidemic impact
and not merely the effectiveness of the intervention in achieving its immediate objectives. A program that achieves statistically significant social
and behavioral changes still may not avert large numbers of new infections. The challenge facing those who allocate prevention resources is to
choose among competing interventions in different locations and to make
decisions about levels of funding. Ideally, decision makers would assess

the efficacy and reach of various interventions against the background of the base rates of infection in different subpopulations. Such analysis would provide tools for predicting the results that might be expected from the many possible options for allocating HIV prevention funds. Today, decision makers virtually never have the information necessary to evaluate either the relative reach and effectiveness of competing programs or the relative risk status of various populations. Even if this information were available, there is no overall agreed upon strategy to guide decision makers' choices.

A STRATEGIC VISION FOR HIV PREVENTION INVESTMENTS

The Committee recommends that CDC and other federal agencies supporting HIV prevention programs adopt a more strategic decision making process for allocating prevention funds. The Committee has already discussed the advantage of allocating funds on the basis of epidemic impact rather than proportionality. Executing that recommendation will require new approaches to deciding which programs to fund and at what levels. Currently, prevention interventions are evaluated based on their individual merit, within an overall allocation based on proportionality. The Committee recommends that funding decisions be made on the basis of maximizing the total number of HIV infections that can be prevented at a given expenditure level. The CDC and other federal agencies should be held accountable for facilitating and managing a funding decision-making process that is guided by that principle. Therefore, the Committee recommends:

> **Prevention resources should be allocated to prevent as many infections as possible. Such an allocation must take into account the cost and effectiveness of programs, in addition to estimates of HIV incidence. Evaluation should be a major component of resource allocation decision making. With better evaluation data reflecting the cost, efficacy, and reach of programs, resources could be more profitably invested in interventions that work efficiently. Interventions that do not work, or that are very expensive relative to infections prevented, could be abandoned.**

While this principle may seem obvious, the Committee found that many current HIV prevention efforts are inconsistent with this goal. The remainder of this chapter describes a resource allocation strategy reflecting this vision, the advantages that would accrue from its use, and some of the problems that must be addressed prior to its implementation.

RESOURCE ALLOCATION FOR HIV PREVENTION

The primary goal of HIV prevention programs should be to prevent HIV infections. Achieving this goal requires prioritizing those combinations of HIV prevention activities that, on the basis of available evidence, are most effective in slowing the spread of disease. However, prevention programs differ in their costs as well as in their effectiveness at slowing HIV transmission. Because there always will be limited resources for HIV prevention, the basic policy and program challenge is how to use available federal funds to support the portfolio of prevention programs that will, in combination, prevent as many new infections as possible.

The Committee believes that allocation decisions regarding public HIV prevention money represent the single most important set of HIV prevention decisions made. The Committee has focused on the number of HIV infections prevented as the best metric for evaluating alternative HIV prevention resource allocation decisions.[7] To the extent that there are additional benefits from these programs (e.g., decreases in drug use or in the incidence of sexually transmitted diseases), the Committee has underestimated total benefits. However, we have also underestimated total costs by focusing only on HIV prevention budgets, whereas funds used for interventions not specific to HIV prevention (e.g., interventions to reduce teen pregnancy) may also reduce HIV infection. This suggests that the resulting allocations could remain reasonable.

The Committee employed a standard model to explore the impact of different allocation decisions. The model, which is described in Appendix D, assumes a societal perspective because it deals with the use of public funds. The examples that follow, developed from the model, illustrate at both a program level and a national level the implications of alternative resource allocation decisions. This analysis assumes a unified HIV prevention budget for purposes of illustrating how different allocation deci-

---

[7]Many analysts prefer to measure effectiveness in units of *quality adjusted life years* (QALYs) instead of infections prevented. Quality adjustments reflect the notion that some health states are preferred to others; a year of healthy life delivers greater utility than a year of disease. The advantage of reporting QALYs is that the cost-effectiveness of HIV interventions (measured in dollars per QALY) becomes comparable to the cost-effectiveness of a host of other interventions ranging from hip replacement surgery to seat belts to diet and exercise regimes to coronary bypass surgery and cancer chemotherapy. The disadvantage, however, is that the assessment of QALYs is by no means straightforward. The degree to which different health states should be discounted relative to perfect health depends on who is doing the discounting as much as on "objective" medical conditions. Since the Committee focuses in this report is confined to HIV prevention, the Committee has adopted the number of HIV infections averted as our effectiveness measure in the review.

sions affect the number of averted HIV infections. In reality, HIV prevention activities—such as counseling and testing, substance abuse treatment, antiretroviral therapy for pregnant women, and school-based HIV prevention education—are financed through separate funding streams, at different levels of government, and within separate organizations that have different organizational philosophies and political constituencies (See Appendix C). The fact that not all programs are funded by the same agency or budget does not invalidate the principle presented. Indeed, the following illustrations demonstrate the importance, given limited resources, of making evidence-based decisions about spending HIV prevention dollars both at the community level and at the national level.

Allocating Resources at the Community Level

As an example, assume that $300,000 will be allocated to programs providing services for injection drug users, and that the programs cost an average of $300 per client. Potentially, 1,000 of an estimated total of 1,500 IDUs in that location could be reached by such an allocation. However, if local conditions are such that only 50 percent of the total IDUs can actually be accessed by the intervention, then only 750 IDUs can be reached by the program—even if funds are available to accommodate 1,000 injectors.

Assume further that, in this location, the annual rate of new infections absent any intervention is equal to five new HIV infections per 100 IDUs per year, and that the program is able to reduce the annual rate of new infections by 20 percent. The result of spending $300,000 would be to reach 750 injectors (since that is the maximum that can be reached), and to reduce the total rate of new infections by 7.5 per year (a reduction from 37.5 to 30 total new HIV infections per year.) Note that 750 IDUs could have been reached by spending only $225,000, implying a misallocation of $75,000.

This example illustrates the problem of allocating the right amount of money to programs for one risk group in one location (Kahn, 1996). The actual challenge of allocating prevention funds across many activities in many locations is far more complex.

Allocating Resources at the National Level

In fiscal year 1999, the CDC distributed approximately $412 million through external cooperative agreements, grants, and contracts for HIV prevention programs nationwide (See Appendix C). To examine how this budget might be allocated to prevent as many infections as possible, the Committee modeled this problem using the same elements as in the previous example. The CDC allocates an HIV prevention budget across dif-

TABLE 3.1 Cost, Reach, and Efficacy of HIV Interventions

Scenario	Injection Drug Users			Men Who Have Sex with Men			Heterosexuals		
	Program Cost per Person	Max. % of Population Reachable	% HIV Incidence Reduction	Program Cost per Person	Max. % of Population Reachable	% HIV Incidence Reduction	Program Cost per Person	Max. % of Population Reachable	% HIV Incidence Reduction
Optimistic	$100	75%	40%	$50	75%	55%	$140	75%	25%
Base	$300	50%	20%	$250	50%	40%	$300	50%	15%
Pessimistic	$700	25%	10%	$500	25%	25%	$500	25%	10%

ferent prevention activities in varied locations. For example, the CDC allocates via the community planning process approximately $258 million to the states, territories, and those large cities hardest hit by HIV/AIDS.

As previously noted, the CDC's HIV prevention funding now follows a pattern of proportionality to AIDS cases. Since AIDS cases appear to be used as a surrogate for HIV incidence when allocating funds, the Committee represents the agency's current policy as proportionality to the rate of new HIV infections. Alternatively, the CDC could allocate funds on the basis of *preventing as many new HIV infections as possible,* within available funding levels. In Appendix D, the Committee details a mathematical model created to solve this problem, and we refer to the results as "cost-effective" allocations. In the model, HIV prevention funds are allocated toward those locations and risk groups in just the right amounts to prevent as many new HIV infections as possible in the aggregate.

The Committee's model can be used to illustrate the improvements that might be gained if the nation invests its resources to prevent the maximum number of new infections. The Committee used this model to examine the impact of proportional policies versus cost-effective allocation policies, and to examine scenarios that assume different levels of investment according to program reach and cost-effectiveness. The model estimates the annual number of new HIV infections prevented at overall budget levels ranging up to $1 billion per year.

To illustrate our case while accounting for the considerable uncertainty in available data, the Committee developed three highly simplified scenarios that bracket the range of possibilities for HIV prevention investments. These are shown in Table 3.1. All are illustrative, as the data describing effectiveness, cost, and reach of programs are very scanty.[8] The scenarios shown were developed on the basis of studies reviewed (see Appendix D for specific references) and against the background of HIV incidence data disaggregated by location and HIV risk group (Holmberg, 1996).[9] The Committee believes that these scenarios provide a plausible illustration of the range of outcomes that the nation might experience under different assumptions of investment levels, program management,

---

[8]See Appendix D for a description of how cost, efficacy, and reach estimates were derived.

[9]The analysis uses estimates of HIV incidence disaggregated by drug injectors, men who have sex with men, and high risk heterosexuals for 96 Standard Metropolitan Statistical Areas in the United States aggregated to the state level (Holmberg, 1996).

and political will to utilize the tools available to confront the epidemic. The three scenarios are:

- *Pessimistic.* Assumes that programs funded have the lowest prevention impact and high costs, and that they reach, on average, 25 percent of the relevant population.
- *Base.* Assumes that programs funded have average effectiveness and average costs, and that they reach 50 percent of the relevant population.
- *Optimistic.* Assumes that programs funded have the largest prevention impact and the lowest costs, and that they reach 75 percent of the relevant population (See Table 3.1).

The figures shown below illustrate that, by shifting investments towards more effective interventions and directing those interventions to the appropriate populations, more new infections can be averted. Figure 3.5 illustrates the impact of each of these scenarios assuming funding levels of up to $1 billion. For each scenario, the upper line reflects epidemic impact using the Committee's recommendation to fund allocation on the basis of estimated HIV infection rates. The lower line illustrates the epidemic impact assuming the current proportional allocation formula. All of the curves exhibit the familiar economic property of diminishing returns to scale: as the amount of money invested in HIV prevention increases, the annual number of infections prevented also increases, but at a decreasing rate. Initial outlays on HIV prevention are thus more beneficial than later outlays.

For each of the three scenarios shown in Figure 3.5, the advantages of cost-effective over proportional allocation are considerable. For example, in the base case, allocating $412 million in proportion to HIV incidence would prevent approximately 3,000 new infections per year. Cost-effective allocation, however, would prevent roughly 3,900 new infections annually, a 30 percent increase.

Note that the proportional policy is worthwhile. Preventing 3,000 infections by spending $412 million yields an average cost of $137,333 per infection prevented, which is not at all unreasonable given that the lifetime medical costs expended for treating HIV infection average near $200,000 per case (Holtgrave and Pinkerton, 1997). However, the cost-effective allocation we propose averts an additional 900 infections for the same $412 million expenditure on prevention.

Figure 3.5 also reveals the value of additional budget increases. Suppose the prevention budget could be increased by 50 percent from $412 to $618 million. In the base case, cost-effective allocation of these resources would enable preventing an additional 540 new infections per year. Com-

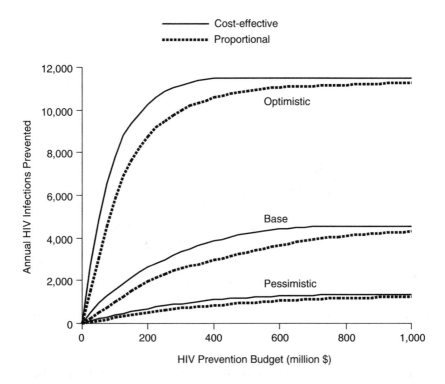

FIGURE 3.5 Annual infections prevented: cost-effective versus proportional allocation.

bining cost-effective allocation with a 50 percent budget increase would thus serve to increase the annual number of infections prevented by nearly 48 percent.

Figure 3.6 illustrates again the advantage to be gained from use of cost-effective rather than proportional allocation strategies. Cost-effective allocation is obviously most important when only limited funds are available; the returns from cost-effective allocations diminish as funds devoted to prevention increase. Nonetheless, in the base and pessimistic scenarios, cost-effective allocation offers at least a 30 percent increase in the number of infections that can be prevented for budgets of $500 million or less.

Against the backdrop of the previous three scenarios, Figure 3.7 shows the return on investments from more research on prevention interventions, with an emphasis on improving both the efficacy and reach of programs that might well be more expensive but that also are more effective. Figure 3.7 illustrates the "investment scenario," whereby the efficacy

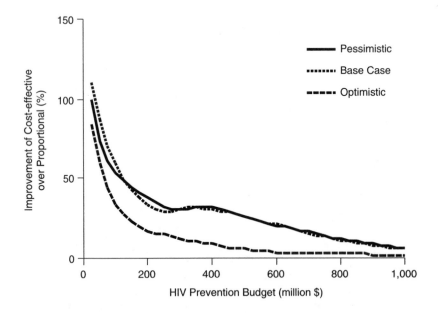

FIGURE 3.6 Cost-effective versus proportional allocation: percentage improvement.

and reach measures are those from the optimistic scenario described in Table 3.1, but costs of prevention per participant are from the pessimistic scenario.

Figure 3.7 makes it clear that investments in prevention can pay off. Assuming optimal allocation, the number of infections that can be prevented in this scenario grows to surpass the base case if at least $100 million is devoted to prevention. This scenario seems a more realistic portrait of what might be expected if investment in improved prevention programs were combined with the cost-effective allocation of prevention funds. At the Committee's touchstone funding level of $412 million, this investment scenario would see the prevention of roughly 5,060 infections under optimal allocation (compared to 3,900 infections prevented in the base case via optimal allocation). The infections averted from proportional spending also would increase modestly from 3,000 in the base case to 3,390 in the investment scenario, again documenting the value of investing in better prevention programs.

The Committee stresses that while these calculations are illustrative, they are sufficiently robust to indicate the very substantial differences in results that could be obtained *at every investment level* by moving toward the recommended principles. While the Committee recommends that fed-

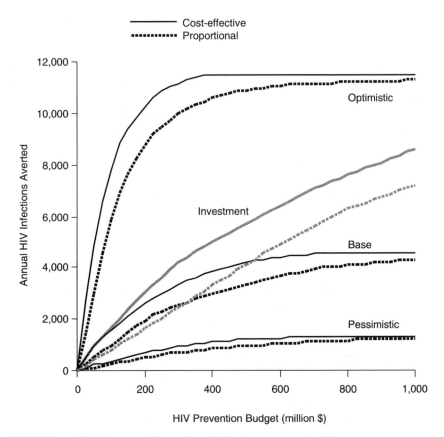

FIGURE 3.7 The impact of investing in better, more expensive programs: cost-effective versus proportional.

eral, state, and local prevention policymakers adopt a cost-effectiveness framework, the Committee is not recommending that federal, state, or local agencies replicate the exact model presented here. Improving the allocation of funds by weighing cost-effectiveness in selecting programs to be funded, and enhancing overall budget levels for prevention programs can effect very meaningful changes in the number of Americans who are infected with HIV. It is important for policy makers to understand the power of these choices and the magnitude of the changes that these choices drive.

The Committee acknowledges that other values will and should play a role in HIV prevention policy. However, it is important that the cost of those values (in terms of prevented HIV infections forgone) be understood and deliberately chosen. Two examples illustrate this point. First, optimal allocations assume that all decisions are driven by the goal of preventing as many new HIV infections as possible, subject to resource constraints. Under certain scenarios (the base case example at $250 million funding, for example), it would not be cost-effective to fund programs aimed at women. Clearly, that would not be an ethical or socially desirable choice. A second example illustrates the cost of placing constraints on available HIV prevention programs based on values that punish socially proscribed behaviors. If needle exchange programs linked to drug treatment were allowed to enter the portfolio of federally funded HIV prevention programs, then the number of new infections prevented at the $412 million investment level is estimated to increase from 3,900 to 5,300 in the base case.[10] The estimated difference of 1,400 prevented infections can be viewed as the human cost imposed by the ban on needle exchange.

SUPPORT FOR STATE AND LOCAL RESOURCE ALLOCATION

The Committee has focused on national-level resource allocation for purposes of illustrating how improved resource allocation can avert more HIV infections. The logic espoused in this chapter applies at the level of state and local governments as well. Implementing a cost-effectiveness decision-making process at the state and local levels, however, poses significant challenges. Two major barriers to conducting economic evaluations at these levels are the lack of technical expertise and the lack of funding. In addition, communities, target populations, and program staff may oppose evaluations out of fear that they will show a program is ineffective or result in a loss of funding. States and localities may also believe that evaluations conducted in other areas are not applicable to their unique needs (Weinstein and Melchreit, 1998). However, the Committee believes that these factors do not detract from the importance of developing a sound foundation for decision making, and the lack of complete information about the costs and benefits of HIV prevention efforts should not deter decision makers at all levels from adopting this framework. Using this framework can also help policy makers formulate a research agenda by pointing to areas where additional data on HIV inci-

---

[10]This estimate follows from combining base case parameters from Table 3.1 for programs targeting men who have sex with men and heterosexuals with the optimistic estimates of program efficacy and reach, but pessimistic costs for programs targeting injection drug users (IDUs). This choice of parameters reflects what might happen if needle exchange programs linked to drug treatment programs were included in the federally funded HIV prevention portfolio.

dence, program costs, and program effectiveness are needed to better inform future decisions.

As the nation's lead prevention agency, the CDC has a special role to play in providing technical assistance to advisory and decision-making bodies at the state and local level on matters regarding the allocation of HIV prevention resources. The CDC's sponsorship of cost-effectiveness workshops at recent community planning national meetings is especially welcomed in this regard. In addition, collaborations and partnerships between federal agencies (including CDC, NIH, SAMHSA, and HRSA), state health departments, community planning groups, and others will be necessary to define a research agenda, to identify and foster expertise for conducting cost-effectiveness studies, and to continue to fund research in cost-effectiveness.

REFERENCES

Anderson RM, May RM. 1991. *Infectious Diseases of Humans: Dynamics and Control.* Oxford, England: Oxford University Press.

AuBuchon JP, Birkmeyer JD, Busch MP. 1997. Safety of the blood supply in the United States: Opportunities and controversies. *Annals of Internal Medicine* 127(10):904–909.

Bayer R. 1997. Science, politics, and AIDS prevention policy. *Journal of Acquired Immune Deficiency Syndromes and Human Retrovirology* 14 (Suppl 2):S22–S29.

Brookmeyer R and Gail MH. 1994. *AIDS Epidemiology: A Quantitative Approach.* New York: Oxford University Press (Monographs in Epidemiology and Biostatistics; v. 22).

Burr C. 1997. The AIDS exception: Privacy vs. Public health. *Atlantic Monthly* 279(6):57–67.

Busch MP, Lee LL, Satten GA, Henrard DR, Farzadegan H, Nelson KE, Read S, Dodd RY, Petersen LR. 1995. Time course of detection of viral and serologic markers preceding human immunodeficiency virus type 1 seroconversion: Implications for screening of blood and tissue donors. *Transfusion* 35(2):91–97.

Carande-Kulis VG, Maciosek MV, Briss PA, Teutsch SM, Zaza S, Truman BI, Messonnier ML, Pappaioanou M, Harris JR, Fielding J. 2000. Methods for systematic reviews of economic evaluations for the Guide to Community Preventive Services. Task Force on Community Preventive Services. *American Journal of Preventive Medicine* 18(1 Suppl):75–91.

Centers for Disease Control and Prevention (CDC). 2000. U.S. Public Health Service Task Force Recommendations for the Use of Antiretroviral Drugs in Pregnant Women Infected with HIV-1 for Maternal Health and for Reducing Perinatal HIV-1 Transmission in the United States. Atlanta: CDC.

Centers for Disease Control and Prevention (CDC). 1999. Provisional Project List by Mission Category for FY99 CDC HIV/AIDS Budget. Atlanta: CDC.

Centers for Disease Control and Prevention (CDC). 1993. Supplemental Guidance on HIV Prevention Community Planning for Non-Competing Continuation of Cooperative Agreements for HIV Prevention Project. Atlanta: CDC.

General Accounting Office (GAO). 2000. Drug Abuse Treatment: Efforts Under Way to Determine Effectiveness of State Programs (GAO/HEHS-00-50). Washington, DC: GAO.

General Accounting Office (GAO). 1998. Blood Plasma Safety: Plasma Products Risks Are Low if Good Manufacturing Practices are Followed. (GAO/HEHS-98-205). Washington, DC: GAO.

General Accounting Office (GAO). 1993. Needle Exchange Programs: Research Suggests Promise as an AIDS Prevention Strategy. (GAO/HRD-93-60). Washington, DC: GAO.

Gold MR, Siegel JE, Russell LB, Weinstein MC (Eds.). 1996. *Cost-Effectiveness in Health and Medicine.* New York: Oxford University Press.

Haddix AC, Teutsch SM, Shafer PA, Dunet DO (Eds.). 1996. *Prevention Effectiveness: A Guide to Decision Analysis and Economic Evaluation.* New York: Oxford University Press.

Health Resources and Services Administration. 2000. The AIDS Epidemic and the Ryan White CARE Act: Past Progress, Future Challenges. Washington, DC: HRSA.

Holmberg SD. 1996. The estimated prevalence and incidence of HIV in 96 large US metropolitan areas. *American Journal of Public Health* 86(5):642–654.

Holtgrave DR (Ed.). 1998. *Handbook of Economic Evaluation of HIV Prevention Programs.* New York: Plenum Press.

Holtgrave DR and Pinkerton SD. 1997. Updates of cost of illness and quality of life estimates for use in economic evaluations of HIV prevention programs. *Journal of Acquired Immune Deficiency Syndromes* 16(1):54–62.

Institute of Medicine. 1999. *Reducing the Odds: Preventing Perinatal Transmission of HIV in the United States.* Stoto MA, Almario DA, and McCormick MC (Eds.). Washington, DC: National Academy Press.

Janssen RS, Satten GA, Stramer SL, Rawal BD, O'Brien TR, Weiblen BJ, Hecht FM, Jack N, Cleghorn FR, Kahn JO, Chesney MA, Busch MP. 1998. New testing strategy to detect early HIV-1 infection for use in incidence estimates and for clinical and prevention purposes. *Journal of the American Medical Association* 280(1):42–48.

Kahn JG. 1996. The cost-effectiveness of HIV prevention targeting: How much more bang for the buck? *American Journal of Public Health* 86(12):1709–1712.

Kahn JG. 1998. Economic Evaluation of Primary HIV Prevention in Injection Drug Users. In Holtgrave DR (Ed.), *Handbook of Economic Evaluation of HIV Prevention Programs.* New York: Plenum Press. Pp. 45–62.

Kaplan EH. 1998. Economic Evaluation and HIV Prevention Community Planning—A Policy Analyst's Perspective. In Holtgrave DR (Ed.), *Handbook of Economic Evaluation of HIV Prevention Programs.* New York: Plenum Press. Pp. 177–193.

Kaplan EH. 1995. Economic analysis of needle exchange. *AIDS* 9(10):1113–1119.

Kaplan EH and Brookmeyer R. 1999. Snapshot estimators of recent HIV incidence rates. *Operations Research* 47(1):29–37.

Kaplan EH and Pollack H. 1998. Allocating HIV Prevention Resources. *Socio-Economic Planning Sciences* 32:257–263.

National Research Council. 1991. *Evaluating AIDS Prevention Programs.* Coyle SL, Boruch RF, and Turner CF (Eds.). Washington, DC: National Academy Press.

National Research Council, Institute of Medicine. 1995. *Preventing HIV Transmission: The Role of Sterile Needles and Bleach.* Normand J, Vlahov D, and Moses LE (Eds.). Washington, DC: National Academy Press.

Petersen LR, Satten GA, Dodd R, Busch M, Kleinman S, Grindon A, Lenes B. 1994. Duration of time from onset of human immunodeficiency virus type 1 infectiousness to development of detectable antibody. The HIV Seroconversion Study Group. *Transfusion* 34(4):283–289.

Phillips KA, Haddix A, Holtgrave DR. 1998. An overview of economic evaluation methodologies and selected issues in methods standardization. In Holtgrave DR (Ed.). *Handbook of Economic Evaluation of HIV Prevention Programs.* New York: Plenum Press.

Stolberg SG. 1998. Clinton decides not to finance needle program. *The New York Times*:A1, April 21.

Substance Abuse and Mental Health Services Administration (SAMHSA). 2000a. HIV Strategic Plan. Washington, DC.: SAMHSA.

Substance Abuse and Mental Health Services Administration (SAMHSA). 2000b. "HIV Designated States" Fiscal Year Obligations, Substance Abuse Prevention and Treatment Block Grant. Washington, DC: SAMHSA.

Teutsch S and Haddix A, (Eds.). 1994. *A Practical Guide to Prevention Effectiveness: Decision and Economic Analysis*. Atlanta: Centers for Disease Control and Prevention.

Valdiserri RO, Aultman TV, Curran JW. 1995. Community planning: A national strategy to improve HIV prevention programs. *Journal of Community Health* 20(2):87–100.

Weinstein B and Melchreit RL. 1998. Economic Evaluation and HIV Prevention Decision Making. In Holtgrave DR (Ed.), *Handbook of Economic Evaluation of HIV Prevention Programs*. New York: Plenum Press.

4

Using the Clinical Setting

The majority of HIV prevention efforts have focused primarily on preventing HIV acquisition by uninfected persons. Several factors conspired to preclude a focus on infected persons, These factors include racism, and homophobia, and the stigma surrounding HIV/AIDS (see Chapter 7 for a more detailed description of these factors). However, given that every new infection begins with someone who already is infected, omitting persons with HIV from prevention efforts represents an important missed opportunity for averting new infections. This failure is made even more glaring by the fact that advances in antiretroviral therapy have considerably increased the number of people living with and receiving care for HIV/AIDS.

It is estimated that 350,000 to 528,000 persons with HIV now make use of the clinical care delivery system and receive regular HIV care (Bozzette et al., 1998). If prevention programs are to more effectively reach those already diagnosed with HIV, then linking clinical care and prevention is a logical next step. Forging this linkage will require that clinical care agencies and providers recognize and act upon their responsibility to provide HIV prevention services, that providers be trained accordingly, and that prevention agencies improve their ties to clinical care.

In this chapter, the Committee describes how existing clinical settings might better integrate HIV prevention activities into their care activities. We also discuss several programmatic and funding changes that may be required to better integrate HIV prevention activities in the clinical care setting.

CLINICAL CARE-BASED PREVENTION

Some guidance on how to integrate HIV prevention into clinical care is available from the U.S. Preventive Services Task Force Guide to Clinical Preventive Services (U.S. Preventive Services Task Force, 1996), which provides a careful review of scientific evidence and indicates which preventive services are most effective. First, the guide recommends that all adolescents and adult patients should be advised about risk factors for HIV and other sexually transmitted diseases (STDs), and counseled about effective measures to reduce the risk of infection. Clinicians are further recommended to assess risk factors for HIV infection by obtaining a careful sexual and drug use history for all patients, and to periodically screen for infection among all persons at increased HIV risk. Providers who care for injection drug users (IDUs) are recommended to advise them about measures to reduce their risk of infection and to refer them to appropriate drug treatment facilities. These basic HIV prevention recommendations become even more critical for clinicians that provide care to patients known to be HIV-infected.

The Committee believes that, in *all* clinical care settings serving HIV-infected persons and those at high risk of infection, the standard of care should include the taking of sexual and drug-using histories to help determine each patient's risk and the appropriate level of HIV prevention intervention. If an HIV-infected individual is found to have another STD, this in itself should trigger the delivery of some type of HIV prevention counseling, as STD infection is a marker for risky sexual behavior. This is particularly important because studies have shown that STDs in an HIV-infected individual may facilitate HIV transmission by increasing the concentration of the virus in genital secretions (Moss and Kreiss, 1990; Cohen et al., 1997).

Even HIV-infected persons receiving antiretroviral therapy can still spread infection. Some studies have shown that antiretroviral therapy can reduce a person's viral load, which has been associated with a decrease in infectiousness of the person's blood or genital secretions (Musicco et al., 1994; Royce et al., 1997; Ragni et al., 1998). These findings suggest the potential use of antiretroviral therapy in HIV prevention. However, a recent study shows that treated individuals may continue to shed HIV even after 6 months of therapy, and thus may continue to pose at least some risk for transmitting the virus to sex partners (Barroso et al., 2000). In addition, recent statistics showing a rise in HIV infections among San Francisco's gay male population (San Francisco Department of Public Health et al., 2000[1]), a community that has high levels of access to antiretroviral therapy, heightens the need to focus prevention interventions on HIV-infected persons and to develop multifaceted approaches to prevention for this population. Furthermore, risky behavior can also compromise the health of the infected person through secondary infections (Blazquez et al., 1995; Cleghorn and Blattner, 1992; Knox and Carrigan, 1995; Phair et al., 1992; Wiley et al., 1993), re-infection with drug-resistant HIV, and such opportunistic infections as tuberculosis (Japour et al., 1995; Johnson, 1995; Larder, 1995).[1]

To build on this initial assessment, clinicians should provide modest but recurring counseling about HIV prevention (including precautions for sexual activity, drug use, and partner notification), in order to reinforce preventive behaviors and assess whether a patient needs more intensive intervention (Francis et al., 1989; Francis, 1996). This type of routine activity within the clinical care setting is perhaps the only means that the public health system has for regularly "checking in" with infected persons about their risk behavior.

Clinicians can also utilize prevention case management techniques to assess risk behavior and reinforce risk reduction among HIV-infected patients. Prevention case management, which is a client-centered, more intensive counseling and risk-management approach to delivering prevention services, has seven essential components: client recruitment and engagement; screening and assessment (comprehensive screening of HIV/STD risks and medical psychosocial service needs); development of a client-centered prevention plan; multiple sessions of HIV risk-reduction counseling; active coordination of services with follow-up; monitoring and reassessment of clients' needs, risks, and progress; and discharge from prevention case management upon attainment and maintenance of risk-reduction goals (CDC, 1997).[2] Prevention case management should also include attention to adherence to HIV antiretroviral therapies to improve and lengthen the lives of those with HIV infection.

Although prevention case management techniques have not been fully evaluated for efficacy and more research is clearly needed, limited results show that these techniques hold promise. For example, the Centers of Disease Control and Prevention and the Health Resources Services Administration sponsored a study of community health centers providing HIV prevention and early intervention services within primary care

---

[1]Recent studies have found that some new cases of HIV infection in untreated patients in which the HIV strain that was transmitted was already resistant to protease inhibitors (Hecht et al., 1998; Dietrich et al., 1999) and reverse transcriptase inhibitors (Fontaine et al., 1998; Brodine et al., 1999). Although the research does not provide conclusive evidence, other data also suggest that reinfection of an already infected individual with other strains of HIV could accelerate HIV disease progression (Angel et al., 2000).

[2]Prevention case management can also be utilized with uninfected, high-risk populations.

programs. Results of this study indicate that HIV-infected persons who received ongoing HIV prevention case management adopted and sustained selected safer sexual practices during the 6 month follow-up period (CDC, 1990). Other studies have found that ongoing counseling can be effective at preventing further transmission, as documented from studying discordant couples[3] (van der Straten et al., 1998, 2000; Sweat et al., 2000; Padian et al., 1993) and in decreasing mother-to-child transmission of HIV (Havens et al., 1997).

In addition to prevention case management, two clinician-delivered HIV prevention interventions are in development for HIV outpatient settings. The "Partnership for Health" study tests three different behavioral interventions for HIV-infected persons (Richardson et al., 2000). Two of the interventions are designed to increase safer sexual behaviors and disclosure of HIV status to sex partners among persons living with HIV using positively versus negatively framed prevention messages about safer sex and disclosure. The third intervention aims to increase antiretroviral treatment adherence; because this intervention does not address sexual behavior, it serves as the comparison (or "control") condition for the safer sex interventions. Six HIV outpatient clinics in California are participating in this study and, upon its completion, health care providers in these clinics will have delivered one or more behavioral interventions to approximately 10,000 HIV-infected persons coming in for care. Preliminary results are expected in 2001 (G. Marks, personal communication). In another study, "Physician Delivered Intervention for HIV+ Individuals," Fisher and colleagues (cited in University of California at San Francisco, 2000) are conducting pilot research for an intervention targeted to clinicians and their HIV-infected clients. The intervention is based on the assumption that many clinicians who provide HIV care are not sufficiently skilled to provide HIV prevention services to their clients. The goal is to develop a physician-directed HIV prevention intervention that can be delivered over time, adapted to meet clients' changing prevention needs, and easily integrated into the context of continuing HIV outpatient care. Preliminary results from this study are expected in 2002 (W. Fisher, personal communication).

Both studies emphasize the role that care providers can play in encouraging adherence to antiretroviral medications and in assessing HIV risk and encouraging safe behaviors. Several studies indicate that a personalized approach by health care providers can optimize patient adherence to antiretroviral therapy by providing careful drug selection in addi-

---

[3]Discordant couples have one HIV-infected partner and one non HIV-infected partner.

tion to routine follow-up and the provision of information, feedback, and reminder systems (Ostrop et al., 2000; Chesney, 2000; Roberts, 2000).

Thus, health care providers play an important role in HIV prevention. Indeed, physicians have been cited by the public as the most trusted source of health information (David and Boldt, 1980), and they are teenagers' preferred source of health information (Manning and Balson, 1989). However, physicians and other providers are often faced with significant barriers to integrating prevention into their standard of care practice. Many clinicians (particularly physicians) may feel that prevention counseling is not within their role of delivering treatment and care, and that these services are best done by other types of health care professionals, such as social workers or counselors (Makadon and Silin, 1995). Although providers' HIV/AIDS knowledge is generally high (Gemson et al., 1991), they may be uncomfortable delivering prevention messages that they feel are ambiguous or confusing (e.g., levels of risk for different types of sexual practices) (Makadon and Silin, 1995). Perhaps the most significant barrier for providers is the lack of comfort or perceived skill in discussing sensitive issues such as substance abuse, sexual behavior, or psychological well-being with patients.

To facilitate the integration of HIV prevention in the care setting, several tools and guides for conducting HIV risk assessments and encouraging safe behaviors have been developed for use by clinical care providers (e.g., Hearst, 1994; American Medical Association, 1996). Also available are predesigned risk assessment algorithms that can guide providers when asking risk-related questions, as well as facilitate discussions about particular aspects of prevention that are most relevant to the patient's risk reduction needs (Cohen, 1995). Such tools and guidelines could be incorporated into current HIV treatment guidelines to ensure that prevention becomes a standard component of clinical care for HIV-infected persons.

Integrating HIV prevention early in health professionals' training and in subsequent continuing education opportunities is another strategy that may improve the skill and comfort level of providers in conducting HIV prevention (Yedidia and Berry, 1999). Such courses could offer training on obtaining sexual and substance use histories, how to deliver clear, effective prevention messages, and how to assist patients in developing realistic risk reduction goals (Makadon and Silin, 1995; Taylor and Moore, 1994; McCance et al., 1991).

HIV testing offers another option for the integration of prevention into the clinical care context. Testing plays multiple roles, including identifying people with HIV and those at risk of infection who can receive prevention services, identifying pregnant women with HIV so they can be offered pharmacological interventions to prevent perinatal transmission, and identifying HIV-infected persons so they can receive more intensive clinical care services (ranging from closer monitoring of immune status to intervention with antiretroviral therapies or prophylaxis for opportunistic infections). The CDC has long maintained the importance of HIV testing as a prevention tool, and recent studies have shown that counseling and testing can be a cost-effective prevention intervention (e.g., Kamb et al., 1998; Weinhardt et al., 1999; The Voluntary HIV-1 Counseling and Testing Efficacy Study Group, 2000).

The CDC also has supported an anonymous HIV counseling and testing infrastructure that is separate from the clinical care setting. Originally created to keep high risk people from using blood banks to learn their HIV status, these alternative testing sites funded by the CDC have often been considered an important part of prevention interventions and a valuable resource for individuals who fear the stigma of HIV testing and want to learn their status in an anonymous setting.

The CDC estimates that 24.6 million people were tested in the United States in 1996. Of these, an estimated 2.6 million tests (not individuals) were performed at CDC publicly funded test sites (CDC, 1998),[4] meaning that the overwhelming majority of HIV tests in 1996 occurred in clinical care settings. If one of the objectives of testing is to identify individuals with HIV and get them into appropriate care (both clinical care and prevention services), the integration of HIV testing services into existing clinical care settings would accomplish several important goals, including assuring that those identified as HIV-infected would have immediate access to clinical care, destigmatizing HIV testing and making it a routine part of care, and promoting the linkage of clinical care and prevention services.

PROGRAMS THAT PROVIDE CLINICAL CARE TO HIV-INFECTED PERSONS

If the clinical care setting is to become a venue for prevention, then it is important to understand where people with HIV are served and how clinical care programs can be better adapted to address prevention needs.

---

[4]The CDC defines its publicly funded sites as those receiving CDC funds; the majority of these sites are clinical care settings but about 26 percent are freestanding counseling and testing sites (CDC, 1990). The CDC definition may exclude HRSA-funded testing sites where a significant number of HIV tests are performed. Community Health Centers (CHCs) alone report performing 218,742 tests in 1998 (National Summary Data, 1999), whereas Title III grantees report performing 315,234 tests in 1997 (HRSA, 1997). This may overlap significantly with the CHC data, since many Title III grantees are CHCs and report to both programs. In addition, many Title III grantees also receive CDC counseling and testing money, and some of these tests might be included in the CDC's data.

HIV/AIDS care is best described as a patchwork of public and private programs. Although little detailed information exists on where HIV-infected persons obtain their health care, two large studies—the AIDS Cost and Services Utilization Survey (ACSUS) (Mohr, 1994) and the HIV Cost and Services Utilization Study (HCSUS) (Frankel et al., 1999)—shed some light on how individuals who know they are HIV-infected use health care services. ACSUS has found that these individuals use health care services in ways similar to the pattern found in the general population in that HIV-infected minorities, females, male IDUs, persons in the lowest income category, and the unemployed are more likely to report a hospital stay or a hospital emergency room visit. In contrast, HIV-infected white persons and those in the highest income category are more likely to visit a private physician's office, use psychological counseling, and use dental care services (Mohr, 1994). The HCSUS notes that most HIV care is provided by a relatively small number of providers. Providers include predominately publicly and privately funded hospitals and clinics, staff or group model HMOs, and private physician or medical groups.

Many people who are HIV-infected but do not know their status seek care from a wide variety of health care settings. For example, young people typically utilize community health centers, drop-in centers, emergency and ambulatory care departments, family planning clinics, and doctors' offices (Steiner and Gest, 1996; Ryan et al., 1996; Hedberg et al., 1996). Women and children with or at risk for HIV/AIDS also rely on a broad array of services from public and private providers. The poor or nearly poor are more likely to use public and nonprofit hospitals, community health centers, family planning clinics, and public health clinics, such as STD clinics (Lyons et al., 1996; Brackbill et al., 1999). In addition, individuals with HIV and those at high risk often have co-occurring substance abuse and mental disorders, and thus receive care from providers in drug treatment centers and mental health clinics. Some segments of the population receive care in specific health care settings, such as the Department of Veterans Affairs Health Care System (VA),[5] the Department of Defense Health Care Systems, and from clinical settings associated with the Department of Justice and state correctional facilities.

Financing of HIV Care

Resources to pay for health care services delivered to HIV-infected persons and those at high risk can also be described as a patchwork of

---

[5]The VA system is the largest single provider of HIV care in the U.S. In 1999, HIV care was provided to 18,000 veterans.

public and private funding streams. Estimates from a nationally representative sample of HIV-infected persons receiving ongoing care found that one-third were covered by private insurance, 29 percent by Medicaid, and 20 percent by Medicare (Bozzette et al., 1998).[6] These estimates varied by race, with a larger percentage of African Americans and Hispanics covered by Medicaid (Bozzette et al, 1998). Many uninsured or underinsured individuals living with HIV also obtain services through the Ryan White CARE Act and Community and Migrant Health Center (CHC) programs, which are administered by HRSA.

Policy initiatives designed to increase the level of prevention offered in clinical care settings can be targeted to private as well as public programs. According to the Health Care Financing Administration (HCFA), Medicaid covers over half of people living with AIDS (HCFA, 2000).[7] Many of these individuals, however, are also eligible for Medicare. CARE Act programs are "payers of last resort" and, therefore, serve primarily low income and indigent populations. Nonetheless, the CARE Act represents the third largest public program paying for care for people living with AIDS, and makes funds available through four titles to states, metropolitan areas, and nonprofit entities. Title I of the Act provides emergency assistance funds to metropolitan areas disproportionately affected by AIDS. Title II provides funds to states to improve the quality, availability, and organization of health care and support services for people with HIV. Title III provides grants to community-based clinics for early intervention services. Title IV provides funds for pediatric AIDS programs (see Appendix C for a more detailed description of CARE Act programs). In fiscal year 2000, CARE Act spending totaled $1.6 billion, compared with an estimated $4.1 billion of federal and state Medicaid HIV/AIDS spending and an estimated $1.7 billion of federal HIV/AIDS Medicare spending (HCFA, 2000). Although the precise number of people served by CARE Act programs is unknown, there may be significant overlap among individuals served by the CARE Act, Medicaid, Medicare, and private insurers.

The Community and Migrant Health Center (CHCs) program is another source of care for people living with HIV. While many CHCs are also HRSA-funded CARE Act grantees, CHCs without CARE Act support are significant providers of federally financed HIV-related primary care to low income populations. In 1998, CHCs conducted over 218,000 HIV

---

[6]Most (80 percent) of the people eligible for Medicare also qualify for Medicaid.

[7]HCFA's estimate is of those with AIDS diagnoses. HCFA has not developed estimates for persons with HIV but not AIDS.

tests, and had over 220,000 HIV-related encounters with infected clients (National Summary Data, 1999). While these are not unduplicated from HIV testing and services that are part of the CARE Act, this remains an impressive number. In parts of the country where there is high HIV incidence and relatively low CARE Act presence (e.g., the rural Southeast), CHCs may be a principal means of reaching and serving those with HIV.

Finally, many HIV-infected persons and those at increased risk receive services from substance abuse treatment and mental health centers. Integrating HIV prevention interventions with the provision of substance abuse and mental health services also can play a critical role in averting new infections. The Substance Abuse Prevention and Treatment Block Grant set-aside for HIV-related services was designed to integrate these services. Although efforts are under way to examine outcomes of these programs, little information is available about how these funds are used or the exact services they provide (GAO, 2000).

CHANGES NEEDED TO ENCOURAGE HIV PREVENTION: MEDICAID AND RYAN WHITE CARE ACT PROGRAMS

If HIV prevention is to be more fully integrated into publicly supported clinical care settings, financing changes are needed to ensure that preventive services are a covered benefit and that these services are adequately reimbursed (Guglielmo, 1999; Makadon and Silin, 1995). This section outlines possible changes to the Medicaid and CARE Act programs that could facilitate the integration of prevention in the clinical care setting.

Financing Options for Medicaid Coverage

There is no mandatory or optional Medicaid service category that specifically covers the components of prevention case management described earlier. However, under the Early and Periodic Screening, Diagnostic, and Treatment program, Medicaid has a mandatory preventive service benefit for children and adolescents under age 21. Additionally, there are two optional service categories that could be used for preventive services for adults with or at high risk for HIV; one of the categories is for screening and preventive services, while the other is for targeted case management services (Committee on Ways and Means, 1998). In order for a benefit to be covered on a fee-for-service basis or through a managed care organization, it must be covered under a state's Medicaid plan and approved by HCFA for federal matching funds.

While the majority (32) of states cover screening and preventive services (Westmoreland, 1999),[8] only 9 state Medicaid programs have opted to cover targeted case management services or counseling for persons with HIV (Jefferys, in press). The targeted case management benefit would permit Medicaid beneficiaries to obtain prevention case management services. Although case management services are applicable to most populations served by Medicaid, states have the option to limit or "target" this benefit to particular subpopulations such as individuals with HIV or AIDS (Schneider and Garfield, 2000). In addition, a state could also choose to target persons considered at high risk for HIV infection, such as persons with sexually transmitted diseases or persons who are addicted to drugs. This benefit can cover services that will assist beneficiaries in gaining access to medical, social, educational, and other services. It is up to the state to establish minimum qualifications for providers offering prevention case management services, which conceivably could include community-based organizations as well as clinical providers.

In order for prevention case management services to be a meaningful service option, HCFA and the CDC need to consider taking a number of steps. HCFA must make clear to state Medicaid agencies that it encourages them to embrace prevention services as part of an HIV-related continuum of care, and that community-based prevention case management, supported through a targeted case management benefit, is one vehicle for achieving this continuum of care. The CDC should work with HCFA and state Medicaid agencies to better define what should be included in this benefit and to assist states in defining the credentials of providers who should be eligible under this benefit. HCFA has issued a number of policy guidances to state Medicaid programs relating to treatment of beneficiaries with HIV and could use this approach to clarify issues regarding prevention services.[9]

States have the option of offering covered services on a fee-for-service basis, through managed care plans, or both. Benefits packages are shaped, in part, by the basis on which they are paid and thus can create financial incentives for the scope and accessibility of these services. Payment systems, therefore, should be considered for the broad implications they might have on whether and how often a covered service is provided.

---

[8]HCFA has by regulation defined "preventive services" as "services provided by a physician or other licensed practitioner ... under state law to (1) prevent disease, disability and other health conditions or their progression, (2) prolong life; and (3) promote physical and mental health and efficiency." C.F.R. 440.130 (c).

[9]See HCFA's website: HtmlResAnchor www.hcfa.gov/medicaid/hiv/hivltrs.htm.

Medicaid Fee for Service. When Medicaid benefits are paid for on a fee-for-service basis, providers recognize that they will be reimbursed only for services that are part of a state's benefit package. Given that there currently is no clearly defined service benefit for some of the major components of preventive case management (e.g., ongoing counseling) that may be required in the context of HIV-related clinical care, it is unlikely that providers will integrate these services into fee-for-service settings until states elect to cover them. States might be encouraged to cover preventive case management services if there were enhanced reimbursement for these services. This would require action by Congress to raise the federal matching rate from the traditional 50 percent to, for example, 90 percent, which is the rate that currently applies in all states to family planning services.[10] In the case of states that currently cover prevention services, they could establish more generous reimbursement rates to encourage practitioners to offer the services. This is action a state could take under current law, with HCFA approval.

Medicaid Managed Care. A state has some flexibility in affecting the delivery of Medicaid covered prevention services through its contract with a managed care organization. The contracting process can be used to integrate covered preventive services into clinical care delivery and require the provision of these services to uninfected individuals at increased HIV risk. There are potential benefits and risks when a managed care organization (MCO) assumes financial responsibility for the care provided. On the one hand, the MCO has a financial incentive to keep patients healthy and thus may be more aggressive about integrating prevention services into clinical care delivery and/or referring clients to appropriate community-based services, using a benefit modeled after the targeted case management benefit. On the other hand, capitation payments can create a financial incentive to withhold approval of services since savings can be applied to the provision of other services. States must take care in contracting with managed care organizations to ensure that the nature of the services expected is clearly defined, that the established managed care networks have the capacity in numbers and expertise to provide these services (including prevention case management), that quality assurance measures hold managed care organizations and their providers accountable for the provision of appropriate prevention services,

---

[10]States receive federal Medicaid matching funds for at least 50 percent and as much as 80 percent of the costs of services for eligible beneficiaries, depending on the average per capita income of the state. Family planning services and supplies are the only exception.

and that capitation rates reflect the expectation that these additional services will be provided.[11]

Encouraging HIV Prevention in CARE Act Programs

While the major premise of the CARE Act is to assure a continuum of services for HIV-infected persons, those services generally have focused on treatment and support services related to primary care. Yet, HIV-infected persons also need prevention services that can help them avoid transmitting the virus to others, as well as prevent their own exposure to opportunistic infections. Such prevention-related services may include HIV prevention interventions and the critically important component of mental health and substance abuse services for those who need them. Without the last element, interventions to prevent the spread of HIV may be much less successful.

The CARE Act does permit grantees to support substance abuse and mental health treatment. However, the only direct mention of prevention in the current law is in the context of preventing perinatal transmission and as part of the pretest counseling offered under Title III. Only Title III is empowered to support outreach to those who have unknown HIV status. The other titles are restricted to serving those already diagnosed with HIV.

Despite numerous provisions in the CARE Act regarding coordination with other service programs, there is only one mention in the current law about coordination with other government agencies involved in prevention. CARE Act grantees are asked to coordinate with the CDC in the context of using surveillance data generated by the CDC (and state and local health departments) for care-related needs assessments. There is no requirement in the legislation that Title I planning councils, Title II consortia, or statewide determinations of need address coordination with government supported prevention initiatives (P.L. 104-146).

HRSA's current regulatory guidance to grantees also minimizes the opportunity to provide prevention services or even coordinate prevention and clinical care services. HRSA has made clear to its grantees that CARE Act funds must be targeted to those who are HIV-infected, not to those who are uninfected but at risk. CARE Act Titles I and II represent the overwhelming majority of CARE Act funding, and they have the most

---

[11]George Washington University's Center for Health Services Research and Policy, under the auspices of CDC and HRSA, has developed *Sample Purchasing Specifications for HIV Infection, AIDS, and HIV-Related Conditions* (August 1999) for use by state Medicaid agencies in purchasing coverage from managed care plans.

flexibility in terms of implementation at the local level. However, the FY2000 guidance documents for both titles make only one mention of prevention in the context of the definition of support services. That definition refers to "health education/risk reduction," which is described as: (1) provision of information, including information dissemination about medical and psychosocial support services and counseling, or (2) preparation/distribution of materials in the context of medical and psychosocial support services to educate clients with HIV about methods to reduce the spread of HIV (HRSA, 1999). These same guidance documents make clear that outreach has as its "principal purpose identifying people with HIV disease so they may become aware of and may be enrolled in care and treatments, *not HIV counseling and testing nor HIV prevention education*" (emphasis added) (HRSA, 1999).

The HRSA guidance also refers to the CDC's syphilis elimination plan, although there is no requirement for coordination. Similarly, the Title I guidance asks grantees to show how they coordinate with prevention planning groups, but there is no requirement that prevention planning groups be included in Title I planning councils, as are representatives of other federally funded programs (HRSA, 2000). The Title II guidance is similarly vague, though states are asked to show their linkages with prevention programs (HRSA, 1999).

HRSA can potentially contribute to more coordinated provision of services with relatively minor modifications of its requirements for Title I and Title II grantees:

- HRSA can require the inclusion of a representative of the prevention planning group on Title I planning councils, on local Title II consortia, and on the group creating statewide coordinated statements of need.
- HRSA can encourage the inclusion of outreach activities to the range of services provided in order to facilitate referral to counseling and testing as well as longer-term prevention services.
- HRSA can encourage all clinical care providers supported by the CARE Act to make HIV risk assessment a standard part of their clinical care encounters in order to judge whether HIV-infected clients are in need of referral to more intensive prevention services.
- As part of the services provided by case managers, HRSA can permit referrals to prevention case management services funded by the CDC (or other agencies), in addition to the current practice of allowing referrals to substance abuse and mental health services. The current definition of case management does not include any reference to coordination with prevention services (HRSA, 2000).

- HRSA can require that its AIDS Education and Training Centers provide training for clinical care providers in undertaking HIV prevention-related activities.

DHHS-WIDE POLICIES TO ENCOURAGE INTEGRATION OF PREVENTION INTO CLINICAL CARE

If the federal government is to fully embrace the goal of integrating prevention services into the clinical care setting, then the government should move to adopt policies that would support the coordination of prevention and care activities at the federal, state, and local levels. Funding policies need particular attention; the current separate funding streams for prevention and clinical care services discourage grantees from integrating these services. The rigid distinction between entitlement and discretionary programs also creates a similar disincentive to bring services together in a "one-stop shopping" approach for people living with or at risk for HIV. Consideration should be given to creating a demonstration program in a series of communities (perhaps using different models) that would allow communities to create integrated systems of clinical care and prevention services by bringing together HIV-related funds from Medicaid, Medicare, HRSA, the CDC, and the Substance Abuse and Mental Health Services Administration (SAMHSA). The outcomes of these demonstration projects will help reveal untoward effects that are not counterbalanced by the potential for administrative efficiencies or by the opportunity to promote greater integration of clinical care and prevention services.

The Committee finds that current prevention programs do not effectively target individuals who are HIV-infected and who may still engage in risky behavior. The Committee believes that all HIV-infected persons should have access to prevention services, and that the clinical care setting provides opportunities for integrating prevention into the standard of care for those who are infected or at high risk. Therefore, the Committee recommends that:

> **Prevention services for HIV-infected persons should be a standard of care in all clinical settings (e.g., primary care settings, sexually transmitted disease clinics, drug treatment facilities, and mental health centers). Health care providers should have adequate training, time, and resources to conduct effective HIV prevention counseling. Enabling this activity may require adjustments in health care provider time allocations and/or specific financial incentives from public and private sources of health coverage.**

REFERENCES

American Medical Association. 1996. Physician Guide to HIV Prevention [Web Page]. Located at: www.hivinsite.ucsf.edu/prevention/guidelines/2098.2751.html.

Angel JB, Kravcik S, Balaskas E, Yen P, Badley AD, Cameron DW, Hu YW. 2000. Documentation of HIV-1 Superinfection and Acceleration of Disease Progression (Abstract LB2). Seventh Conference on Retroviruses and Opportunistic Infections; Jan 31–Feb 2, 2000; San Francisco.

Barroso PF, Schechter M, Gupta P, Melo MF, Vieira M, Murta FC, Souza Y, Harrison LH. 2000. Effect of antiretroviral therapy on HIV shedding in semen. *Annals of Internal Medicine* 133(4):280–284.

Blazquez MV, Madueno JA, Jurado R, Fernandez-Arcas N, Munoz E. 1995. Human herpesvirus-6 and the course of human immunodeficiency virus infection. *Journal of Acquired Immune Deficiency Syndromes and Human Retrovirology* 9(4):389–394.

Bozzette SA, Berry SH, Duan N, Frankel MR, Leibowitz AA, Lefkowitz D, Emmons CA, Senterfitt JW, Berk ML, Morton SC, Shapiro MF. 1998. The care of HIV-infected adults in the United States. HIV Cost and Services Utilization Study Consortium. *New England Journal of Medicine* 339(26):1897–1904.

Brackbill RM, Sternberg MR, Fishbein M. 1999. Where do people go for treatment of sexually transmitted diseases? *Family Planning Perspectives* 31(1):10–15.

Brodine SK, Shaffer RA, Starkey MJ, Tasker SA, Gilcrest JL, Louder MK, Barile A, VanCott TC, Vahey MT, McCutchan FE, Birx DL, Richman DD, Mascola JR. 1999. Drug resistance patterns, genetic subtypes, clinical features, and risk factors in military personnel with HIV-1 seroconversion. *Annals of Internal Medicine* 131(7):502–506.

Centers for Disease Control and Prevention (CDC). 1990. Publicly funded HIV counseling and testing—United States, 1985–1989. *Morbidity and Mortality Weekly Report* 39(9):137–140.

Centers for Disease Control and Prevention (CDC). 1997. HIV Prevention Case Management: Literature Review and Current Practice. Atlanta, CDC.

Centers for Disease Control and Prevention (CDC). 1998. HIV Counseling and Testing in Publicly Funded Sites: 1996 Annual Report. Atlanta: CDC.

Chesney MA. 2000. Factors affecting adherence to antiretroviral therapy. *Clinical Infectious Diseases* 30 (Suppl) 2:S171–176.

Cleghorn FR and Blattner WA. 1992. Does human T-cell lymphotropic virus type I and human immunodeficiency virus type 1 coinfection accelerate acquired immunodeficiency syndrome? The jury is still out. *Archives of Internal Medicine* 152(7):1372–1373.

Cohen MS. 1995. HIV and sexually transmitted diseases. The physician's role in prevention. *Postgraduate Medicine* 98(3):52–58, 63–64.

Cohen MS, Hoffman IF, Royce RA, Kazembe P, Dyer JR, Daly CC, Zimba D, Vernazza PL, Maida M, Fiscus SA, Eron, JJ Jr. 1997. Reduction of concentration of HIV-1 in semen after treatment of urethritis: Implications for prevention of sexual transmission of HIV-1. AIDSCAP Malawi Research Group. *Lancet* 349(9069):1868–1873.

Committee on Ways and Means. U.S. House of Representatives. 1998. *1998 Green Book: Background Material and Data on Programs within the Jurisdiction of the Committee on Ways and Means.* (WMCP-105-7) Washington, DC: U.S. Government Printing Office.

David A and Boldt JS. 1980. A study of preventive health attitudes and behaviors in a family practice setting. *Journal of Family Practice* 11(1):77–84.

Dietrich U, Raudonat I, Wolf E, Jager H, Husak R, Orfanos CE, Knickmann M, Knechten H, von Briesen H, Ruppach H, Immelmann A. 1999. Indication for increasing prevalence of resistance mutations for protease inhibitors in therapy-naive HIV-1-positive German patients. *AIDS* 13(16):2304–2305.

Fisher, W. The University of Western Ontario, Department of Obstetrics and Gynaecology. Personal communication, September 13, 2000.

Fontaine E, Lambert C, Servais J, Ninove D, Plesseria JM, Staub T, Arendt V, Kirpach P, Robert I, Schneider F, Hemmer R, Schmit JC. 1998. Fast genotypic detection of drug resistance mutations in the HIV-1 reverse transcriptase gene of treatment-naive patients. *Journal of Human Virology* 1(7):451–456.

Francis DP. 1996. Every person infected with HIV-1 should be in a lifelong early intervention program. *Sexually Transmitted Diseases* 23(5):351–352.

Francis DP, Anderson RE, Gorman ME, Fenstersheib M, Padian NS, Kizer KW, Conant MA. 1989. Targeting AIDS prevention and treatment toward HIV-1-infected persons. The concept of early intervention. *Journal of the American Medical Association* 262(18):2572–2576.

Frankel MR, Shapiro MF, Duan N, Morton SC, Berry SH, Brown JA, Burnam MA, Cohn SE, Goldman DP, McCaffrey DF, Smith SM, St. Clair PA, Tebow JF, Bozzette SA. 1999. National probability samples in studies of low-prevalence diseases. Part II: Designing and implementing the HIV cost and services utilization study sample. *Health Services Research* 34(5 Part 1):969–992.

Gemson DH, Colombotos J, Elinson J, Fordyce EJ, Hynes M, Stoneburner R. 1991. Acquired immunodeficiency syndrome prevention. Knowledge, attitudes, and practices of primary care physicians. *Archives of Internal Medicine* 151(6):1102–1108.

General Accounting Office (GAO). 2000. *Drug Abuse Treatment: Efforts Under Way to Determine Effectiveness of State Programs* (GAO/HEHS-00-50). Washington, DC: GAO.

Guglielmo WJ. 1999. Why more doctors aren't testing for HIV. *Medical Economics* 76(11):180–182, 187–188, 191–192 *passim*.

Havens PL, Cuene BE, Hand JR, Gern JE, Sullivan BW, Chusid MJ. 1997. Effectiveness of intensive nurse case management in decreasing vertical transmission of human immunodeficiency virus infection in Wisconsin. *Pediatric Infectious Disease Journal* 16(9):871–875.

Health Care Financing Administration. 2000. Medicaid and Acquired Immune Deficiency Syndrome and Human Immunodeficiency Virus Infection [Web Page]. Located at: www.hcfa.gov/medicaid/obs11.htm.

Health Resources and Service Administration, HIV/AIDS Bureau, Division of Service Systems. 1997. Title III 1997 Program Data Report, Executive Summary [Web Page]. Located at: www.hrsa.gov/hab/data.html.

Health Resources and Services Administration, HIV/AIDS Bureau, Division of Service Systems. 1999. The Ryan White Comprehensive AIDS Resources Emergency (CARE) Act: Title II HIV CARE Grant Program, FY 2000 Grant Application Guidance for States. Rockville, MD: HRSA.

Health Resources and Services Administration, HIV/AIDS Bureau, Division of Services Systems. 2000. The Ryan White Comprehensive AIDS Resources Emergency (CARE) Act: Title I HIV Emergency Relief Grant Program, FY 2001 Grant Application Guidance. Rockville, MD: HRSA.

Hearst N. 1994. AIDS risk assessment in primary care. *Journal of the American Board of Family Practice* 7(1):44–48.

Hecht FM, Grant RM, Petropoulos CJ, Dillon B, Chesney MA, Tian H, Hellmann NS, Bandrapalli NI, Digilio L, Branson B, Kahn JO. 1998. Sexual transmission of an HIV-1 variant resistant to multiple reverse transcriptase and protease inhibitors. *New England Journal of Medicine* 339(5):307–311.

Hedberg VA, Byrd RS, Klein JD, Auinger JD, Weitzman M. 1996. The role of community health centers in providing preventive care to adolescents. *Archives of Pediatric Adolescent Medicine* 150(6):603–608.

Japour AJ, Welles S, D'Aquila RT, Johnson VA, Richman DD, Coombs RW, Reichelderfer PS, Kahn JO, Crumpacker CS, Kuritzkes DR. 1995. Prevalence and clinical significance of zidovudine resistance mutations in human immunodeficiency virus isolated from patients after long-term zidovudine treatment. AIDS Clinical Trials Group 116B/117 Study Team and the Virology Committee Resistance Working Group. *Journal of Infectious Diseases* 171(5):1172–1179.

Jefferys, R. In press. Survey of State Medicaid Programs on HIV/AIDS. Menlo Park: CA. AIDS Treatment Data Network/Kaiser Family Foundation.

Johnson VA. 1995. Nucleoside reverse transcriptase inhibitors and resistance of human immunodeficiency virus type 1. *Journal of Infectious Diseases* 171 (Suppl 2):S140–149.

Kamb ML, Fishbein M, Douglas JM, Rhodes F, Rogers J, Bolan G, Zenilman J, Hoxworth T, Malotte CK, Iatesta M, Kent C, Lentz A, Graziano S, Byers RH, Peterman TA. 1998. Efficacy of risk reduction counseling to prevent human immunodeficiency virus and sexually transmitted disease: A randomized controlled trial. *Journal of the American Medical Association* 280(13):1161–1167.

Knox KK and Carrigan DR. 1995. Active human herpesvirus (HHV-6) infection of the central nervous system in patients with AIDS. *Journal of Acquired Immune Deficiency Syndrome and Human Retrovirology* 9(1):69–73.

Larder BA. 1995. Viral resistance and the selection of antiretroviral combinations. *Journal of Acquired Immune Deficiency Syndromes and Human Retrovirology* 10 (Suppl 1):S28–33.

Lyons B, Salganicoff A, Rowland D. 1996. Poverty, Access, and Health Care, and the Medicaid's Critical Role for Women. In Falik MM and Collins KS (Eds.), *Women's Health: The Commonwealth Survey*. Baltimore, MD: Johns Hopkins University Press.

Makadon HJ and Silin JG. 1995. Prevention of HIV infection in primary care: Current practices, future possibilities. *Annals of Internal Medicine* 123(9):715–719.

Manning D and Balson P. 1989. Teenagers' beliefs about AIDS education and physicians' perceptions about them. *Journal of Family Practice* 29(2):173–177.

Marks G. Centers for Disease Control and Prevention. Personal communication, July 14, 2000 and September 14, 2000.

McCance KL, Moser R Jr, Smith KR. 1991. A survey of physicians' knowledge and application of AIDS prevention capabilities. *American Journal of Preventive Medicine* 7(3):141–145.

Mohr P. 1994. Patterns of health care use among HIV-infected adults: Preliminary results. *ACSUS Report* 3:1–19.

Moss GB and Kreiss JK. 1990. The interrelationship between human immunodeficiency virus infection and other sexually transmitted diseases. *Medical Clinics of North America* 74(6):1647–1660.

Musicco M, Lazzarin A, Nicolosi A, Gasparini M, Costigliola P, Arici C, Saracco A. 1994. Antiretroviral treatment of men infected with human immunodeficiency virus type 1 reduces the incidence of heterosexual transmission. Italian Study Group on HIV Heterosexual Transmission. *Archives of Internal Medicine* 154(17):1971–1976.

National Summary Data. 1999. Bureau of Primary Health Care Uniform Data System, National Summary Data 1998. MDS Associates and Stickold Associates.

Ostrop NJ, Hallett KA, Gill MJ. 2000. Long-term patient adherence to antiretroviral therapy. *Annals of Pharmacotherapy* 34(6):703–709.

Padian NS, O'Brien TR, Chang Y, Glass S, Francis DP. 1993. Prevention of heterosexual transmission of human immunodeficiency virus through couple counseling. *Journal of Acquired Immune Deficiency Syndromes* 6(9):1043–1048.

Phair J, Jacobson L, Detels R, Rinaldo C, Saah A, Schrager L, Munoz A. 1992. Acquired immune deficiency syndrome occurring within 5 years of infection with human immunodeficiency virus type-1: The Multicenter AIDS Cohort Study. *Journal of Acquired Immune Deficiency Syndromes* 5(5):490–496.

Public Law 104-136. A compilation of the Ryan White CARE Act of 1990, as amended by the Ryan White CARE Act amendments of 1996.

Ragni MV, Faruki H, Kingsley LA. 1998. Heterosexual HIV-1 transmission and viral load in hemophilic patients. *Journal of Acquired Immune Deficiency Syndromes and Human Retrovirology* 17(1):42–45.

Richardson JL, Stoyanoff SR, Bolan R, Kemper C, Hollander H, Larsen R, Weismuller P, Weiss JM, McCutchan A. Brief safer sex intervention for HIV outpatient clinics (Poster # TuPeD3660). XIII International AIDS Conference; Jul 9–Jul 14, 2000; Durban, South Africa.

Roberts KJ. 2000. Barriers to and facilitators of HIV-positive patients' adherence to antiretroviral treatment regimens. *AIDS Patient Care STDs* 14(3):155–168.

Royce RA, Sena A, Cates W Jr, Cohen MS. 1997. Sexual transmission of HIV. *New England Journal of Medicine* 336(15):1072–1078.

Ryan SA, Millstein SG, Greene B, Irwin CE Jr. 1996. Utilization of ambulatory health services by urban adolescents. *Journal of Adolescent Health* 18(3):192–202.

San Francisco Department of Public Health, AIDS Research Institute, University of California, San Francisco. 2000. Response to the Updated Estimates of HIV infection in San Francisco, 2000.

Schneider A and Garfield R. 2000. *Medicaid Benefits* (Report #2150). Washington, DC: The Kaiser Commission on Medicaid and the Uninsured.

Steiner BD and Gest KL. 1996. Do adolescents want to hear preventive counseling messages in outpatient settings? *Journal of Family Practice* 43(4):375–381.

Sweat M, Gregorich S, Sangiwa G, Furlonge C, Balmer D, Kamenga C, Grinstead O, Coates T. 2000. Cost-effectiveness of voluntary HIV-1 counselling and testing in reducing sexual transmission of HIV-1 in Kenya and Tanzania. *Lancet* 356(9224):113–121.

Taylor WC and Moore GT. 1994. Health promotion and disease prevention: Integration into a medical school curriculum. *Medical Education* 28(6):481–487.

U.S. Preventive Services Task Force. 1996. Guide to Clinical Preventive Services, 2nd Edition. Washington, DC: U.S. Department of Health and Human Services.

University of California at San Francisco. 2000. Primary prevention for people living with HIV. AIDS Research Institute Monograph.

van der Straten A, Vernon KA, Knight KR, Gomez CA, Padian NS. 1998. Managing HIV among serodiscordant heterosexual couples: Serostatus, stigma and sex. *AIDS Care* 10(5):533–548.

van der Straten A, Gomez CA, Saul J, Quan J, Padian N. 2000. Sexual risk behaviors among heterosexual HIV serodiscordant couples in the era of post-exposure prevention and viral suppressive therapy. *AIDS* 14(4):F47–54.

Voluntary HIV-1 Counseling and Testing Efficacy Study Group. 2000. Efficacy of voluntary HIV-1 counseling and testing in individuals and couples in Kenya, Tanzania, and Trinidad: A randomised trial. *Lancet* 356:103–112.

Weinhardt LS, Carey MP, Johnson BT, Bickham NS. 1999. Effects of HIV counseling and testing on sexual risk behavior: A meta-analytic review of the published research, 1985–1997. *American Journal of Public Health* 89(9):1397–1405.

Westmoreland T. 1999. Medicaid and HIV/AIDS Policy: A Basic Primer. Washington, DC: Kaiser Family Foundation and Federal Legislation Clinic of Georgetown University Law Center.

Wiley DJ, Visscher B, Detels R, Murphy R. 1993. Gonorrhea and syphilis infection as risk factors for short-term rapid CD4+ decline in a cohort of HIV-infected men who have sex with men (Abstract 179). First National Conference of Human Retroviruses and Related Infections; Dec 12–16, 1993; Washington, DC.

Yedidia MJ and Berry CA. 1999. The impact of residency training on physicians' AIDS-related treatment practices: a longitudinal panel study. *Academic Medicine* 74(5):532–538.

5

Translating Research into Action

Avariety of interventions are available for preventing HIV infections (see Appendix B). Many of these interventions emphasize changing risk behaviors related to sexual practices or drug use, under the assumption that the adoption of "safer" behaviors will reduce individuals' risk of exposure to (and infection with) HIV. Other interventions rely on technological approaches to preventing HIV transmission. Although research and clinical trials can evaluate the efficacy of these interventions, the true test of whether or not they are useful for HIV prevention is how well they actually function in community or "field" settings. In order for the interventions to make the transition from the research setting to the field setting, they must be "transferred"—that is, disseminated and adopted—to community-based organizations (CBOs), AIDS service organizations (ASOs), and other groups that can implement them on a local level.

In this chapter, the Committee examines the efforts that have been made in transferring prevention technologies, and we present testimony by community members about the usefulness and effectiveness of these efforts. The Committee also provides recommendations for how technology transfer can be improved.

CURRENT EFFORTS IN PREVENTION TECHNOLOGY TRANSFER

Over the years, the National Institutes of Health (NIH), Centers for Disease Control and Prevention (CDC), and other federal agencies have funded social and behavioral research that has yielded interventions that significantly reduce HIV-related risk behavior, thereby reducing HIV infection risk. Although such research projects are valuable for the development of better social and behavioral prevention tools, their findings typically have been disseminated in a very select manner (e.g., peer-reviewed articles) via very select mechanisms (e.g., clinical or academic journals and conferences) to a very select audience (e.g., other researchers). This strategy is effective in reaching mainly academic audiences, but it is ineffective in disseminating the methodologies and findings to those who need them the most: state- and local-level workers who are planning, developing, adapting, and implementing prevention activities in their communities.

In recognition of the need for greater dissemination of prevention technologies, the Presidential Advisory Council on HIV/AIDS (PACHA) recommended in 1996 that the President "should instruct the Secretary of Health and Human Services to ensure that federally funded research on HIV prevention interventions include specific mechanisms for rapid dissemination of findings, including resources to allow replication of programs with demonstrated effectiveness" (PACHA, 1996). To address this, the CDC responded that its Prevention Research Synthesis (PRS) project—which, at that time, was already in development—would meet the recommended objective. The PRS project created an ongoing database of HIV prevention interventions that were selected for their methodological rigor and that had substantial evidence of effectiveness. Additionally, the PRS project was charged with developing mechanisms for the dissemination and adoption of these interventions. For example, the project led to the development of the Compendium of HIV Prevention Interventions with Evidence of Effectiveness (CDC, 1999a), the Characteristics of Reputationally Strong Programs Project (CDC, 2000b), and the CDC Behavioral and Social Science Volunteer Project (CDC, 2000a). The CDC and various partners also have provided technical assistance to support the implementation of science-based prevention.

These and other vehicles for improving access to research also have been developed by federal and private agencies and are available to the general public. Examples of these methods are presented in Table 5.1.[1]

Each of the resources listed in Table 5.1 provides brief descriptions of specific prevention interventions, including information about their meth-

---

[1]The Committee did not conduct a systematic review of the technical assistance activities offered by the CDC and other organizations. This table illustrates the kinds of technical assistance currently offered.

TABLE 5.1 Examples of HIV Prevention Research Dissemination

Authors	Title	Description of Interventions	Dissemination Tool
CDC/NCHSTP (CDC, 2000d)	REP+: Replicating Effective Programs Plus http://www.cdc.gov/hiv/projects/rep/default.htm	Science-based, tested behavioral interventions with demonstrated evidence of effectiveness in reducing HIV risk behaviors	Intervention packages/kits
CDC/NCHSTP (CDC, 1999a)	Compendium of HIV Prevention Interventions with Evidence of Effectiveness http://www.cdc.gov/hiv/projects/rep/compend.htm	Prevention interventions that have been tested in research settings, have shown no negative findings, and have yielded statistically significant changes in HIV risk behavior	Document
CDC/NCHSTP (CDC, 2000b)	C-RSP Project: Characteristics of Reputationally Strong Programs http://www.cdc.gov/hiv/projects/rep/crspproj.htm	Prevention programs that are "well-respected" and "reputationally strong," but that have not been evaluated by research trials and are seldom published	Document

CDC/NCCDPHP-DASH (CDC, 2000c)	Programs that Work http://www.cdc.gov/nccdphp/dash/rtc/hiv-carric/htm	HIV prevention programs specifically designed for use in adolescent and school-based populations	Curricula and fact sheets
NASTAD, AED, CDC (NASTAD et al., 2000)	Bright Ideas: Innovative or promising practices in HIV prevention and HIV prevention community planning http://www.cdc.gov/hiv/pubs/brightideas.pdf	A compilation of innovative state-level prevention (and community planning) activities that "jurisdictions' peers felt were notable"	Document
Sociometrics Program Archives	Program Archive on Sexuality, Health, and Adolescence (PASHA) http://www.socio.com/pasha/poview.htm	"A collection of promising teen pregnancy and STD/HIV/AIDS prevention programs for teens"	Intervention packages/kits for sale
Sociometrics Program Archives	HIV/AIDS Prevention Program Archive (HAPPA) http://www.socio.com/pasha/happa.htm	"A collection of promising adult HIV/AIDS prevention programs"	Intervention packages/kits for sale

SOURCE: CDC: Centers for Disease Control and Prevention; NCSTP: National Center for HIV, STDs, and TB Prevention; NCCPDHP-DASH: National Center for Chronic Disease Prevention and Health Promotion, Division of Adolescent and School Health; NASTAD: National Alliance of State AIDS Directors; AED: Academy of Educational Development

odologies, target audiences, and program effects (e.g., significant changes in risk behavior). Further, each resource lists whom to contact to obtain more information about the interventions, and each of them is available via the Internet. In some cases (e.g., the Sociometrics Program Archives), ready-made intervention "kits" are available for purchase for those wishing to adopt interventions in school, group, or community settings. In many cases, these kits have been adapted so that the materials and curricula are user-friendly and written in language appropriate for local-level use. In addition to the resources listed in Table 5.1, the CDC Behavioral and Social Science Volunteer Project links technical prevention science volunteers with local prevention providers for the purpose of helping to build intervention research and implementation skills.

State and local level health departments can also offer technical assistance to community organizations (NASTAD, 2000a). Indeed, health departments are in a good position to provide coordinated assistance and capacity development to community prevention service providers because they have access to infected and at-risk communities, as well as access to relevant federal agencies. Additionally, because they are federally mandated to provide such assistance, health departments are more likely to have the necessary infrastructure in place to effectively provide support to community-level colleagues (NASTAD, 2000a).

BARRIERS TO EFFECTIVE TECHNOLOGY TRANSFER AT THE COMMUNITY LEVEL

Despite the above-mentioned efforts, community representatives (ranging from state health department officials to outreach workers) reported to the Committee that the actual level of technology transfer and technical assistance being offered by both federal, state, and local agencies is not enough to help them address "real world" prevention needs (see Appendix E for summary of public comments). Although the representatives acknowledged and appreciated the efforts that have been made by the CDC and other federal agencies that fund prevention activities, they generally felt that the technical assistance being delivered is insufficient in terms of quantity and occasionally variable in quality. Several representatives expressed a need for technical assistance to improve the organizational capacity of CBOs and ASOs so that they could successfully support prevention services for their constituents. According to these representatives, the lack of organizational capacity is, in some cases, due to insufficient personnel resources at the organization and the need for more staff to help manage the increases in workload that come with the adoption of new prevention programs. In other cases, the general lack of information from technical assistance providers regarding the type of infrastructure needed for implementation of new prevention programs precluded the organization from being able to assess where their own organizational capacity was lacking. Some representatives also expressed a need for technical advisers who would spend significantly more time at their site (e.g., one to two weeks) to get better acquainted with the service-providing organization and the prevention needs of the targeted risk groups, as well as to help the organization muster support from the community. The representatives felt that, with a deeper understanding of the local context, technical specialists could provide more useful advice regarding the organizational and implementation-related problems that occur on a day-to-day basis.

With regard to current efforts, some representatives believed that the intervention dissemination process is too slow to keep up with the social and behavioral risk trends that continue to occur in the highest risk communities. Some representatives also said that social and behavioral interventions that are too heavily focused on theory are not practical or culturally relevant when applied at the field level, and that disseminating "interventions in a box" does not work without resources to aid adaptation and implementation. And some representatives stressed the need for building local-level capacity so that CBOs and ASOs could design their own interventions that would be both scientifically sound and better suited to the prevention needs and realities of their constituencies. It was felt that such capacity building could be done on a "peer-to-peer" basis using local community experts or through improved, egalitarian collaborations with research groups and state health departments.

It also was clear from the testimony of the community representatives that other important information, skills, and methodologies are not being effectively disseminated to the field. For example, many representatives cited difficulty in obtaining current data regarding the effectiveness of programs, including cost-effectiveness, for prevention interventions. Some representatives pointed out the need for valid, reliable evaluation methodologies, as well as for training on their use, to evaluate both the effectiveness and cost-effectiveness of prevention programs that could be used at the local level by health departments, CBOs, and others to better estimate the true impact of the interventions on the HIV infection rates in their communities. It also was felt that such information could provide better guidance for choosing the right interventions to suit both constituents' needs and local operating budgets. Because the continuation of funding for state and local prevention services often depends on some indication of the program's effectiveness, the absence of such data or the methodology with which to collect these data has potentially serious consequences for the continuity of HIV prevention services in a given community.

Lastly, many community representatives cited issues related to funding as obstacles to optimal implementation and maintenance of prevention services. For example, several representatives specifically mentioned that the prevention and care needs of individuals diagnosed with multiple disorders could be better served if organizations were better provided with technical assistance on obtaining and sustaining funding for prevention services. Such assistance could take the form of training in grant writing, or guidance regarding how to use merged funding streams to provide complementary HIV prevention services (e.g., substance abuse treatment and HIV prevention outreach) that are supported through different federal agencies. Such technical assistance could be provided at the state and local levels by liaisons from federal agencies and through closer collaborations with research organizations and health departments.

The views expressed by the community representatives are not new. Such views have been documented in the research literature (Stevenson and White, 1994) and in community public forums (Goldstein and Lew, 1998). Also, the Presidential Advisory Council, in its 1997 response to the Clinton Administration's actions regarding its technology transfer recommendation, stated that although it was pleased with the CDC's development of a program concerning technology transfer, "The Council lacks sufficient information to evaluate the effectiveness of this program" (PACHA, 1997). The Council added that, in general, the federal effort in this area "falls well short of what is needed to ensure that local prevention service providers have access to the latest prevention research findings." The 1999 Work Group Report on HIV Prevention Activities at the CDC, submitted to the CDC Advisory Committee for HIV and STD Prevention (ACHSP), echoed the call for more effective mechanisms for disseminating prevention technologies, recommending that the CDC "develop a technical assistance process that drives a real technology transfer agenda" (CDC, 1999b). The report further noted that "technical assistance is NOT technology transfer."

OPPORTUNITIES FOR IMPROVING PREVENTION TECHNOLOGY TRANSFER

There are several key mechanisms by which the transfer and adaptation of prevention research can occur in a more timely fashion. At the state and local levels, one way in which prevention technologies can be more effectively transferred to and implemented by communities is through the establishment of additional collaborative partnerships between prevention researchers (who are often based in universities) and local prevention service providers (Shriver et al., 1998; Sanstad et al., 1999; Schensul, 1999). These collaborations can facilitate the development of program evaluations and new interventions that are more realistic and culturally appropriate to the communities to which the interventions are targeted (Grinstead et al., 1999; Klein et al., 1999). Such partnerships may initially be difficult to forge because of perceived power differentials, differences in social class, and trust issues. To be successful these partnerships must be egalitarian, mutually respectful, and bi-directional in their level of information exchange (Schensul, 1999).

An example of such a partnership is the Center for AIDS Prevention Studies (CAPS) model of community-based collaborative research at the University of California, San Francisco (Sanstad et al., 1999; Schensul, 1999). Created and initiated in 1991 in response to National Institute of Mental Health's (NIMH) mandate for community involvement as a condition for receiving funding, the underlying goal of the CAPS model is to bring the skills of science to the service of HIV prevention and the knowledge of the service providers into the domain of research. This model has been applied in two different programs, one that is limited to the Bay Area[2] and one that is statewide.[3] Process and outcome evaluations of these programs indicate that they have improved interorganizational communication and increased the value of research for service providers, and that, in some cases, their research findings have influenced policy at the agency level in terms of service delivery (Schensul, 1999).

Compared to national organizations, state and local research centers that are funded by NIH agencies (such as the National Institute for Drug Abuse and the NIMH) are ideally suited to help implement technology transfer. They are not only able to provide research expertise, but also are able to provide continuing consultation and on-site technical assistance to the CBOs implementing prevention interventions. Given that such federally funded centers exist throughout the country, they have the opportunity to form regional networks of technology transfer centers that can work with communities to address the HIV epidemic as it manifests itself in those locations. This sort of active collaboration has been shown to result in more successful adoption of science-based prevention programs

---

[2]The program in the San Francisco Bay Area is the HIV Prevention Evaluation initiative. Managed by CAPS, the initiative brings together CBOs, CAPS researchers, CAPS program administrators, and area philanthropists to implement HIV prevention intervention research (Sanstad et al., 1999). For more information about this program, see: http://www.caps.ucsf.edu/capsweb/ncgindex.html.

[3]The Statewide Community HIV Evaluation Project consists of researcher-CBO teams located throughout California, who implemented formative and outcome research (Sanstad et al., 1999). For more information about this program, see: http://www.caps.ucsf.edu/capsweb/projects/schepindex.html.

at the community level (Kelly et al., 2000), and such collaboration also has been shown to be a contributing factor to successful community-based research overall (Goldstein et al., 2000). Although the CAPS model has been replicated by universities, funding agencies, and CBOs nationally (Goldstein et al., 2000), the testimony submitted by community representatives to the Committee regarding the need for ongoing, more comprehensive technical assistance and research collaborations suggests that this mechanism for technology transfer is still underutilized.

At the federal level, there are several opportunities for improving prevention research technology transfer. For example, the CDC has extensive interaction with prevention service providers at the state and local levels and it already provides a substantial amount of technical assistance to community-based organizations. Given this established role on the "front lines" of prevention, the CDC should evaluate the quality and quantity of technical assistance that it has provided in order to determine how the process can be improved. For example, a 1996 report on the CDC's HIV Prevention Community Planning Process found that there was limited incorporation of behavioral research into community planning (Collins and Franks, 1996). Some of the barriers included the lack of group training on the use of behavior research; questions about the applicability of the research to specific at-risk populations or geographic areas; gaps in the behavioral research literature; and widely divergent levels of planning group members' expertise, education, and familiarity with research information (Collins and Franks, 1996).

While the CDC is the lead prevention agency, other agencies in the Department of Health and Human Services also have a substantial role in the national HIV prevention effort, and their roles can be expanded. For example, while the 18 NIH-funded Centers for AIDS Research (CFARs) currently have a mandate of "facilitating technology transfer and development through promotion of scientific interactions between CFARs and industry," (NIH, 1995), this mission could be expanded to include more active collaborations between CFARs specializing in prevention research and non-industry organizations, such as state and local health departments and community-based HIV prevention service providers. Similarly, the NIMH's Center for Mental Health Research on AIDS, which supports basic and applied behavioral research on HIV prevention (NIH, 1999), could expand its mission to include greater support of research pertaining to the dissemination and adaptation of effective prevention interventions into community settings. Such actions were called for in the 1996 Report of the NIH AIDS Research Program Evaluation Working Group of the Office of AIDS Research Advisory Council, which urged NIH "to continue to support HIV community involvement in AIDS research programs" (Office of AIDS Research Advisory Council, 1996). The report further stated that "translating basic laboratory and behavioral sciences research into public health and clinical practice is an essential aspect of a (AIDS Research) Center's program that can in turn, provide further basic research opportunities" (Office of AIDS Research Advisory Council, 1996).

Because NIH supports a significant amount of research activities related to HIV prevention, it might be the agency best suited to investigate ways to better disseminate and adapt prevention technologies to the community level. Such efforts should be undertaken in collaboration with partner agencies which have a large role in local-level prevention efforts, such as the CDC, the Substance Abuse and Mental Health Services Administration, and the Health Resources and Services Administration.

Based on this evidence, the Committee acknowledges that, without greatly improved HIV prevention dissemination and adoption mechanisms and associated technical assistance, the organizations that operate HIV prevention programs at the state and local levels will continue to struggle against the obstacles that limit their effectiveness. Therefore, the Committee recommends:

Key Department of Health and Human Services agencies that fund HIV prevention research and interventions should invest in strengthening local-level capacity to develop, evaluate, implement, and support effective programs in the community. The Committee further recommends that these agencies invest in research on how best to adapt effective programs for use in community-level interventions and research on what constitutes effective technical assistance for optimal research-to-community transfer of prevention programs; these agencies should also be responsible for the widespread dissemination of the results of this research. Such efforts will require the participation and collaboration of the funding agencies, researchers, service providers, and communities.

REFERENCES

Centers for Disease Control and Prevention (CDC), Prevention Research Synthesis Project. 1999a. Compendium of HIV prevention interventions with evidence of effectiveness. Atlanta, CDC.

Centers for Disease Control and Prevention (CDC). (Work Group on HIV Prevention at the CDC). 1999b. Final report to the Advisory Committee on HIV and STD Prevention. Atlanta, CDC.

Centers for Disease Control and Prevention (CDC). 2000a. Behavioral and Social Science Volunteer Program [Web Page]. Located at: www.cdc.gov/hiv/projects/rep/bssv. htm.

Centers for Disease Control and Prevention (CDC). 2000b. The C-RSP Project: Characteristics of Reputationally Strong Programs [Web Page]. Located at: www.cdc.gov/hiv/projects/rep/crspproj.html.

Centers for Disease Control and Prevention (CDC). 2000c. Programs that Work: HIV Prevention Curriculum and Fact Sheets [Web Page]. Located at: www.cdc.gov/nccdphp/dash/rtc/hiv-curric.htm.

Centers for Disease Control and Prevention (CDC). 2000d. Replicating Effective Programs Plus [Web Page]. Located at: www.cdc.gov/hiv/projects/rep/default.htm.

Collins C and Franks P. 1996. Improving the use of behavioral research in the CDC's HIV prevention community planning process: Centers for AIDS Prevention Studies, University of California, San Francisco. Monograph Series, Occasional Paper #1.

Goldstein E, Freedman B, Richards A, Grinstead O. 2000. The legacy project: Lessons learned about conducting community-based research [Web Page]. Located at: www.caps.uscf.edu/bibindex.html#S2C.

Goldstein E and Lew S. 1998. New Directions in Prevention. Presentation. Mayor's Summit on AIDS and HIV, San Francisco, CA [Web Page]. Located at: hivinsite.uscf.edu/social/misc._documents/2098.3723.html.

Grinstead OA, Zack B, Faigeles B. 1999. Collaborative research to prevent HIV among male prison inmates and their female partners. *Health Education and Behavior* 26(2):225–238.

Kelly JA, Somlai AM, DiFranceisco WJ, Otto-Salaj LL, McAuliffe TL, Hackl KL, Heckman TG, Holtgrave DR, Rompa D. 2000. Bridging the gap between the science and service of HIV prevention: Transferring effective research-based HIV prevention interventions to community AIDS service providers. *American Journal of Public Health* 90(7):1082–1088.

Klein D, Williams D, Witbrodt J. 1999. The collaboration process in HIV prevention and evaluation in an urban American Indian clinic for women. *Health Education and Behavior* 26(2):239–249.

National Alliance of State and Territorial AIDS Directors. 2000a. Technical assistance and capacity building provided to community based organizations by health departments. *NASTAD Issue Briefs.*

National Alliance of State and Territorial AIDS Directors, Academy of Educational Development, Centers for Disease Control and Prevention. 2000b. Bright Ideas: Innovative or Promising Practices in HIV Prevention and HIV Prevention Community Planning [Web Page]. Located at: www.cdc.gov/hiv/pubs/brightideas.pdf.

National Institutes of Health. 1995. Centers for AIDS Research (CFAR) Mission Statement (developed by the CFAR Directors at the 1995 Annual Directors Meeting) [Web Page]. Located at: www.niaid.nih.gov/research/cfar/Mission2.htm.

National Institutes of Health. 1999. Overview of the Mission of the Center for Mental Health Research on AIDS [Web Page]. Located at: www.nimh.nih.gov/oa.

Office of AIDS Research Advisory Council.1996. Report of the NIH AIDS Research Program Evaluation Working Group of the Office of AIDS Research Advisory Council [Web Page]. Located at: www.nih.gov/od/oar/public/public.htm.

Presidential Advisory Council on HIV/AIDS. 1996. PACHA recommendations—unresolved only. Council Recommendation III.P.4. Washington DC: PACHA.

Presidential Advisory Council on HIV/AIDS. 1997. PACHA recommendations—unresolved only. Council Assessment of Response III.P.4. Washington DC: PACHA.

Sanstad KH, Stall R, Goldstein E, Everett W, Brousseau R. 1999. Collaborative community research consortium: A model for HIV prevention. *Health Education and Behavior* 26(2):171–184.

Schensul JJ. 1999. Organizing community research partnerships in the struggle against AIDS. *Health Education and Behavior* 26(2):266–283.

Shriver M, de Burger R, Brown C, Simpson HL, Meyerson B. 1998. Bridging the gap between science and practice: insight to researchers from practitioners. *Public Health Reports* 113 (Suppl 1):189–193.

Sociometrics. HIV/AIDS Prevention Program Archive (HAPPA) [Web Page]. Located at: www.socio.com/pasha/happa/htm.

Sociometrics. Program Archive on Sexuality, Health, and Adolescence (PASHA) [Web Page]. Located at: www.socio.com/pasha/poview.htm.

Stevenson HC, White JJ. 1994. AIDS prevention struggles in ethnocultural neighborhoods: Why research partnerships with community based organizations can't wait. *AIDS Education and Prevention* 6(2):126–139.

6

Searching for New Tools

There are a number of biomedical and technological advances that, with continued development and expanded use, may help in HIV prevention efforts. These advances include rapid testing methods for detecting HIV antibodies and providing same-day results, female condoms, microbicides, antiretroviral therapies, and vaccines. Two of these technologies (rapid-testing methods and female condoms) already are available but are not widely used in the United States, and two of them (microbicides and vaccines) are still in the development phase. Antiretroviral therapies are known to be effective in preventing HIV transmission from perinatal and occupational exposures, but their wider use for prevention is still largely undetermined.

In this chapter, the Committee discusses the promise that these technologies offer for preventing new HIV infections, and we describe how development of these technologies can be accelerated by increased collaboration among public and private-sector agencies.

PROMISING NEW TOOLS

Rapid Testing Methods for Detecting HIV Antibodies

The Centers for Disease Control and Prevention (CDC) recently estimated that as many as 275,000 individuals in the United States are not aware that they are infected with HIV (CDC, 2000b). Knowing one's HIV status is a critical component of prevention. HIV testing, combined with appropriate counseling, can be an effective strategy for encouraging individuals to adopt risk-reduction behaviors, either to maintain their uninfected status or to prevent transmitting infection to others (e.g., Kamb et al., 1998; Weinhardt et al., 1999; The Voluntary HIV-1 Counseling and Testing Efficacy Study Group, 2000). Because the counseling and testing experience combines diagnostic technology with human interaction, it also offers important opportunities to provide personalized risk-reduction advice and assistance with partner notification, and those who test positive can be linked with needed medical care and social-support services.

Studies conducted in publicly funded testing sites reveal that, on average, approximately two-thirds of individuals tested return to learn their test results and receive post-test counseling (CDC, 1996). One study, for example, found that approximately 26 percent of the individuals tested who turned out to be infected and 33 percent of those who were found to be uninfected did not return for their test results (CDC, 1998). While the return rates may vary by population (e.g., Rotheram-Borus et al., 1997; Valdiserri et al., 1993), the fact remains that a substantial number of people never return to know their HIV status. With standard HIV testing procedures that use an enzyme immunoassay (EIA), there is a one-week to two-week period between the drawing of blood for the test and the availability of the test result.[1] Other new HIV tests that use standard diagnostic methodologies for nonplasma fluids (e.g., whole blood, urine, and oral fluid samples) also require approximately one to two weeks to obtain results (Kassler, 1997).

Given the increasing percentage of people who are getting tested for HIV infection (from 18 percent in 1987 to 40 percent in 1995) (Anderson et al., 2000), new testing options that encourage more people to obtain their results may expand the number of individuals who know their status. In contrast, rapid HIV tests deliver results in approximately 10 minutes, enabling health care workers to provide results[2] and post-test counseling in the same visit (CDC, 1998). Although several rapid tests have been developed, the Single Use Diagnostic System (SUDS) test is the only such test that is approved by the Food and Drug Administration (FDA) for use

---

[1]The time lapse with these methods of testing occurs because tests are generally processed in batches in order to decrease testing costs, and because time is needed to conduct confirmatory testing of reactive EIA tests (Kassler, 1997).

[2]A positive rapid-test result is considered a "preliminary positive," as it has not yet been confirmed using a Western Blot test or immunofluorescence assay. Individuals testing positive would be told of the need for confirmatory testing, but would still be given post-test counseling as if receiving a positive test result (Kassler, 1997).

in the United States, and is comparable to the standard EIA in terms of diagnostic accuracy (Kassler et al., 1995). Rapid tests have also been developed for whole blood and oral fluid samples and home collection HIV test kits, but have not yet been approved by the Food and Drug Administration (Kassler, 1997).

Evidence suggests that rapid testing is feasible, accepted by clients, and may significantly increase the proportion of individuals who learn their HIV status (Kassler et al., 1997; Irwin et al., 1996). Because the entire testing and counseling experience is conducted in the same day, rapid tests can enable health care workers to take full advantage of the "teachable moments" that may occur when, by requesting HIV testing, individuals are psychologically more open to prevention education and can benefit from information about treatment services. Rapid testing may be particularly useful in prenatal care and labor and delivery settings (Grobman and Garcia, 1999), as well as in the case of occupational exposure (Kassler, 1997), where information about HIV status is needed to make immediate decisions about the initiation of antiretroviral therapies to reduce the risk of HIV infection. Studies also suggest that rapid testing may be useful in urban hospital emergency departments (Kelen et al., 1999; Kelen et al., 1995), which remain primary sources of care for many individuals who are at risk of HIV infection (Solomon et al., 1998; Lindsay et al., 1993). Another advantage of rapid tests is that they can be easily employed in nonclinical settings, thereby expanding the capacity of outreach and other community-based prevention settings that serve populations (e.g., the homeless or injection drug users) who may not have consistent access to health care services (Kassler, 1997).

Despite the advantages, there are concerns about using rapid tests to convey positive results on the same day without a confirmatory test. For example, significant emotional anxiety can result from having to wait for a preliminary positive result of a rapid test to be confirmed by a standard diagnostic test, such as a Western Blot. However, recent studies in developing countries indicate that combinations of rapid antibody assays (e.g., using tests made by different manufacturers) are effective in providing accurate confirmatory results in a timely manner (e.g., Stetler et al, 1997; Meda et al., 1999; Andersson et al., 1997). Further, there is evidence to suggest that clients prefer rapid testing methodologies and prefer receiving their results on the same day that they are tested (Kassler et al., 1997). These findings underscore the need for expedited approval and licensing of other rapid tests so that this methodology can be more widely and more confidently used in outreach and other settings where rapid testing would be appropriate and acceptable.

There also are concerns about the potential for using coercion to use rapid testing methodologies to test individuals for HIV antibodies without their consent. For example, should rapid, easy to use blood or saliva tests become readily available to the public, the chances might be increased that unwilling individuals would be forced to submit to testing at home or when applying for jobs (Vanchieri, 1996). For these reasons, it is important to ensure that statutory protections against discrimination and testing without informed consent (similar to protections discussed in the federal Americans with Disabilities Act) are enforced, and, if necessary, that additional protective legislation be enacted (Bayer et al., 1995).

Additionally, there are concerns about the cost of rapid tests; the SUDS test costs about $10, whereas standard EIA tests cost approximately $2.50 (Kane, 1999). However, a study of the use of rapid testing for pregnant women in labor who did not have prenatal care indicated that the cost savings generated by the reduction in perinatal HIV transmission (achieved by giving therapeutic zidovudine to women found to be infected) outweighs the higher testing costs; in this case, the result was a total cost savings to the U.S. medical system of $6 million per year per 100,000 women presenting without adequate prenatal care (Grobman and Garcia, 1999). Another study in an urban emergency room setting also found significant cost savings from the use of rapid testing methodologies (Kelen et al., 1999).

Alternative Barrier Methods

The development of chemical and physical barriers that can be used intravaginally or intrarectally to prevent the acquisition of HIV and other sexually transmitted diseases (STDs) is critically important to the control of HIV infection. The development of alternative barrier products is especially important because of the increasing prevalence of heterosexual transmission of HIV worldwide and the recognized inability or unwillingness of women to insist that their partners use male condoms. These alternative barrier products also can be used by men who have sex with men. Two barrier methods under development seem especially promising: the female condom and microbicides.

The Female Condom

The male latex condom, when used consistently and correctly, can reduce the chances of HIV acquisition by more than 95 percent (e.g., Davis and Weller, 1999; Pinkerton and Abramson, 1997). Indeed, condom use currently is the most effective way of preventing sexual transmission of HIV (Pinkerton and Abramson, 1997; Weller, 1993) and is a key element of most HIV prevention programs. However, male condoms typically are used only at the discretion of the male partner. Although the female condom has a level of efficacy comparable to other barrier methods for preventing pregnancy and STDs (Soper et al., 1993; Trussell et al., 1994), it has not yet been studied for efficacy in preventing HIV transmission specifically. Still, because these polyurethane devices are 40 percent stronger than latex condoms and have been demonstrated in laboratory studies to be virtually impenetrable to viral leakage (Elias and Coggins, 1996), their prospects for preventing HIV transmission seem good (Elias and Coggins, 1996; Soper et al., 1993).

Although the female condom has been on the market for a number of years and is used in some developing countries (e.g., Madrigal et al., 1998; Musaba et al., 1998), its use in the United States is still quite limited. In a number of trials in the United States, the condoms have generally received favorable ratings of acceptability among heterosexual women (e.g., Witte et al., 1999; El-Bassel et al., 1998; Klein et al., 1999; Farr et al., 1994; Shervington, 1993), heterosexual men (e.g., Seal and Ehrhardt, 1999; El-Bassel et al., 1998; Klein et al., 1999), and men who have sex with men (Gibson et al., 1999), but other factors make it a less acceptable alternative to male condoms. One of the major obstacles is its price, which ranges from $2 to $4 per condom, thus making it a less affordable alternative to male condoms[3] (Forbes, 1997). Additionally, because the female condom is still a visually noticeable method of protection, partners who are reluctant to use any barrier method may object to this method as well. Other obstacles to wider usage include lack of familiarity with the device and insufficient knowledge of where to obtain it (e.g., McGill et al., 1998). More aggressive social marketing strategies may be able to increase the future utilization of the female condom for HIV prevention.

Microbicides

Microbicides act as chemical barriers to prevent the transmission of HIV and other STDs. The development of such agents is one of the world's greatest prevention needs because a microbicide is the only current HIV prevention tool that can be used by women who lack the power or willingness to negotiate condom use with male partners. Microbicides represent a true user-controlled method that can be employed without the consent of a sexual partner.

Microbicides use several methods to prevent HIV infection, including blocking the virus from entering mucosal cells (e.g., Neurath et al., 1996; Pearce-Pratt and Phillips, 1996; Miller et al., 1995), killing or inactivating

---

[3]According to a 1997 article, Medicaid coverage in most states will pay for the purchase of female condoms if they are prescribed by a physician (Forbes, 1997).

the virus (e.g., Thompson et al., 1996; Voeller and Anderson, 1992; Redondo-Lopez et al., 1990), or preventing viral replication (e.g., Van Damme and Rosenberg, 1999; Lawson et al., 1999). The ideal microbicide would be easy to use; tasteless, colorless, and odorless; effective against a range of sexually transmissible pathogens (including HIV); nontoxic; stable in a variety of climates; allow for reproductive function; and afford-able (Lawson et al., 1999; International Working Group on Vaginal Micro-bicides, 1996). Development of a microbicide product that meets all these criteria, however, poses significant technological challenges.

The only topical microbicides now available are contraceptive sperm-icides. The most widely used spermicide is nonoxynol-9 (N-9), a deter-gent that destroys microbial cell membranes. N-9 has a protective effect against some STDs (e.g., d'Oro et al., 1994) and, in laboratory studies, has been shown to have a protective effect against HIV (Bird, 1991; Malkovsky et al., 1988). However, evidence is mixed regarding the effectiveness of N-9 against HIV when used in practical situations. Some studies have sug-gested that N-9 has a protective effect, while others have found that N-9 users have an increased risk of HIV infection (perhaps due to genital irritation that could facilitate HIV transmission) (Roddy et al., 1998a; Feldblum et al., 1995). Further evidence against N-9 comes from a major microbicide trial in which the study group using N-9 was found to have a higher rate of infection that the group using a placebo (Van Damme, 2000). Other studies have found no effect against HIV (Roddy, 1998b). Given the conflicting evidence and the incomparability of trial data due to variations in type and amount of N-9 used, the Centers for Disease Con-trol and Prevention recommends that N-9 should not be used for HIV prevention (CDC, 2000a).

In addition to the technological challenges faced in developing effec-tive topical microbicides, there are challenges to conducting clinical trials to evaluate their efficacy. For example, the use of a placebo may be prob-lematic because it may adversely affect vaginal flora. In addition, stan-dard ethical protocols in microbicide clinical trials require the use of condoms by all trial subjects, which makes it difficult to distinguish whether significant protective effects are due to the condom or the micro-bicide (Lawson et al., 1999; Wulf et al., 1999; de Zoysa et al., 1998).

Thus, there remains an urgent need to develop effective anti-HIV microbicides. There are numerous preventive microbicides in various stages of development: 36 products are in preclinical trials, 20 are ready for human safety trials, and three are under consideration for Phase III safety and efficacy trials (UNAIDS, 2000). But researchers estimate that it will still be several years before any of these products can be approved for use (Lawson et al., 1999), mainly because work on microbicide develop-ment is significantly under-funded. The Alliance for Microbicide Development estimates that an investment of $100 million per year over the next five years will be necessary to develop an effective microbicide (Population Council and International Family Health, 2000). However, since 1996, the United States has invested only approximately $25 million to $30 million in microbicide research (Wulf et al., 1999; Population Council and International Family Health, 2000), while philanthropic sources have contributed approximately $6–$10 million (Heise, 2000). Although it is anticipated that an effective microbicide will be available prior to a vaccine for HIV (UNAIDS, 2000), efforts for microbicide development, testing, and licensure should be accelerated so that these products can be made available to consumers in both developing and developed countries. The prioritization of microbicide research and development will require increased levels of funding and the removal of barriers, such as the lack of private-sector investment. These issues will be discussed in greater detail later in this chapter.

Antiretroviral Therapies

Since the introduction in 1985 of the first antiretroviral drug, zidovudine, dramatic advancements have been made in developing stronger and more effective antiretroviral agents to treat HIV infection. With 15 antiretroviral drugs now available and more in development (e.g., fusion inhibitors, which prevent the virus from entering and inserting its genetic material into the host cell) (Stephenson, 2000), HIV infection is quickly becoming a chronic, manageable condition.

It is now common practice for HIV-infected persons to take combinations of antiretroviral drugs. Recent evidence indicates that such combination treatment is effective in reducing the viral load of infected individuals to an undetectable level which, in turn, often results in a variety of favorable health outcomes (e.g., halted disease progression, improvements in CD4+ lymphocyte counts, and increased survival time) (Collier et al., 1996; Gulick et al., 1997; Deeks et al., 1997). Lowered viral load also has been associated with a decrease in infectiousness of the person's blood or genital secretions (Musicco et al., 1994; Royce et al., 1997; Ragni et al., 1998). Further, there is strong evidence that lowered viral concentration in an HIV-infected mother's blood greatly reduces the risk of perinatal transmission (IOM, 1999; Connor et al., 1994).

In addition to these findings, a recent study in Africa found that no viral transmission occurred from infected partners to uninfected partners (via sexual intercourse) when the infected person had less than 1,500 copies of the virus per millimeter of blood plasma (Quinn et al., 2000). These findings are of particular interest because the HIV-infected persons were not using antiretroviral therapies. Given the ability of these drugs to reduce viral load significantly and the evidence pertaining to reduced viral burden in the genital secretions of infected persons on antiretoviral therapies, there is great promise that similar protective effects against sexual transmission of HIV can be obtained using antiretroviral therapies. However, this promise must be balanced with caution. The effectiveness of combination antiretroviral therapies is thought to have contributed to a resurgence in risk behavior among men who have sex with men, due to their perception that HIV infection is no longer a significant health threat (Kelly et al., 1998a; Kelly et al., 1998b; Dilley et al., 1997). Other studies of gay men and HIV-infected men and women suggest that reductions in viral load associated with antiretroviral therapies may prompt individuals to believe that seropositive sexual partners who are taking these medications are less infectious (Kalichman et al., 1998; Kravcik et al., 1998), particularly if they also had an undetectable viral load (Vanable et al., 2000). As there are no data yet specifically to support these hypotheses, more research is needed to determine the benefits that these treatments may have for HIV prevention.

Vaccines

The development of a protective vaccine for HIV infection has been a primary goal since the beginning of the HIV/AIDS epidemic. Research has focused on developing both a preventive vaccine, which would prevent infection or prevent development of symptoms in those infected but asymptomatic, and a therapeutic vaccine, which would slow or stop progression of disease in infected, symptomatic individuals.

Despite significant advances in understanding of the virus, its biology, and its interaction with the human body, fundamental scientific and economic barriers hinder the development of a human vaccine for HIV. First, there are no adequate animal models in which to test the efficacy of vaccines prior to use in humans; available models are either too costly or inadequately mimic human infection and the disease processes. Second, the nature of the immune response needed to prevent HIV is unknown, as there have been no cases of recovery that can be studied. Third, the vaccines under development are primarily oriented toward clade B, the strain of the virus that is most common in wealthier nations (Kremer, 2000a). Given the significant genetic diversity among clades, it is uncertain whether a vaccine that proves effective for one clade would provide protection against different viral subtypes (Kimball et al., 1995; Lawson et al., 1999).

Economic incentives to encourage private sector investment in HIV vaccine research also are lacking due to factors such as the general underconsumption of vaccines (particularly by developing nations with limited health care resources) and the unwillingness of private industries to pursue research and development opportunities that are socially valuable or which contribute to the international public good (Berkley, in press; Kremer, 2000a). Vaccine research and development is considered commercially very risky; it is expensive and time consuming, taking approximately 10–12 years to develop a new product and bring it to market (Berkley, in press). Further, vaccine research and development often does not yield a significant financial return on investment, as it often takes more than a decade for companies to recover their research and development costs for a new vaccine (Berkley, in press; Kremer, 2000a). Although private investment in vaccine development has improved, most companies have relegated such work to a lower priority due to the higher demand and market for therapeutic drugs (e.g., antiretrovirals), as well as the length of time required for product development, testing, and approval (Kimball et al., 1995). As a result, most of the investments in HIV vaccine research have come from the public sector (IAVI, 2000). The International AIDS Vaccine Initiative (IAVI) and other organizations are currently spearheading efforts to encourage more private sector investment in vaccine research and development (IAVI, 2000).

Nevertheless, some candidate vaccines have shown promise in protecting against HIV infection and have been tested in humans. Trials of vaccines derived from viral subunits (i.e., genetically engineered proteins of HIV) suggest that they provide only a limited protective response (Berman et al., 1997; Schwartz et al., 1993). However, in recognition of the fact that a vaccine that generates any amount of protective response may help in curtailing the epidemic in the developing world, where it is most acute, efficacy trials of subunit vaccines are currently under way in Thailand and Uganda. Vaccine trials using live attenuated HIV are being seriously considered, but have not yet been conducted in humans due to safety concerns. Other vaccine strategies, including using live virus vector and DNA vaccines, are currently being investigated (Berkley, in press; Lawson et al., 1999). Issues of greatest concern in vaccine trials include the safety and immunogenicity of vaccines, their effectiveness against infection and disease resulting from different modes of transmission, and the permanence of the protective response (Lawson et al., 1999).

Similarly, there is concern that availability of a vaccine that is even partially effective could contribute to resurgences in risk behaviors (Blower and McLean, 1994). To curb the potential adverse effects, prior to vaccine clinical trials or immunization programs, prevention and education programs must be implemented and sustained to ensure that behaviors to prevent HIV transmission are continued (Lawson et al., 1999). Even when a vaccine is available, it would be important to maintain emphasis on and invest in other prevention efforts (e.g., counseling and testing, risk reduction education, provision of barrier methods, etc.) that could be provided simultaneously with a vaccine to prevent other sexually transmitted infections or unwanted pregnancies (Berkley, in press).

The characteristics of the virus, including its high mutability, its different modes of transmission, and the differing biological characteristics of its affected populations make the development of a universally effective vaccine problematic. Given these factors, it will be essential to discourage perceptions that a vaccine is a "magic bullet" that will forever eliminate HIV.

PROMISING NEW COLLABORATIONS

While new technologies have much to offer to HIV prevention, there are significant barriers to the timely development, approval, and distribution of such innovations. These barriers include insufficient funding to maintain research on product development and testing and lack of interest on the part of pharmaceutical companies and other public/private sector agencies to invest in the development of the product.

Consider the development of microbicides. Most of the research and development efforts to advance microbicidal products are conducted by academic, federal, and biotechnology company laboratories. While these efforts have produced approximately 59 microbicide products that currently are in various stages of clinical testing, N-9 has been the only microbicide that has become available throughout the course of the epidemic. The reason for the lack of microbicidal options lies primarily with the lack of interest and involvement on the part of the pharmaceutical industry and other private-sector groups that have the experience and resources, as well as the manufacturing and marketing skills, to bring promising microbicide candidates to market (Blakeslee, 2000). A 1996 Medical Research Council survey of 13 medium and large-sized international pharmaceutical companies identified three main reasons for their hesitation to invest in microbicides. Foremost was the lack of definitive clinical evidence of microbicide efficacy. Another concern was the difficulty of developing a product that has a high enough degree of efficacy to satisfy regulatory agencies, yet has characteristics that are acceptable to consumers (e.g., tasteless, odorless, easy to use). Further, companies were concerned about the lack of convincing evidence of a profitable market for microbicides. Other reasons included the potential poor return on investment, the cost and duration of the development process, the prospect of litigation, difficulties in obtaining patents, and the probability of having to work cooperatively with the public sector (Blakeslee, 2000). A subsequent survey of 30 pharmaceutical companies found that, while many of these concerns had waned due to increased evidence for marketability and efficacy, only four of the 30 firms expressed willingness to become involved in microbicide development (Blakeslee, 2000).

Despite new efficacy and acceptability data, the concern about product profitability remains. This concern has affected the level of research surrounding a variety of other diseases, particularly those (e.g., tuberculosis and malaria) that primarily affect the impoverished and socially disadvantaged in both developed and developing countries. Two major reports, the 1990 Report of the Commission on Health Research for Development and the 1996 report of the WHO Ad Hoc Committee on Health Research, concluded that of the $56 billion spent on health research annually, less than 10 percent is directed toward the diseases that affect 90 percent of the world's population (cited in Global Forum for Health Research, 1999). Given that developing countries bear an estimated 95 percent of the global HIV/AIDS burden and have the greatest need for preventive products, research on microbicides (as well as on vaccines) certainly falls into this category.

Increased concern about the market's failure to respond to diseases of the poor has led to the development of public/private partnerships that foster innovation in research for such diseases. The International AIDS Vaccine Initiative, created in 1995, and the Alliance for Microbicide Development and the Consortium for Industrial Collaboration in Contraceptive Research, both created in 1999, are examples of such partnerships. Philanthropic and private organizations—such as the William and Flora Hewlett Foundation, the Moriah Fund, the Bill and Melinda Gates Foundation, and the American Foundation for AIDS Research—recently have begun to contribute to microbicide research. Additionally, the World Bank has announced that it will "ensure the availability of funds to purchase and distribute microbicides to developing countries once they become available," in an effort to guarantee market viability and provide incentives to pharmaceutical companies to invest in microbicide research (Mitchell, 2000).[4]

These partnerships are a promising start to the promotion of microbicide development. Similar collaborations are needed to advance the development of other preventive technologies. The timely development of these products will require the prioritization of research efforts and the promotion of public/private sector collaborations. Additionally, to increase involvement by private sector industries (e.g., pharmaceutical companies) and philanthropic sources, there is a great need for the development of economic incentives, such as vaccine purchase commitments (Berkley, in press; Kremer, 2000b), "push-pull" initiatives to encourage

---

[4]A similar initiative was created by the World Bank for HIV vaccine research.

greater industry participation (Berkley, in press), tiered pricing mechanisms (i.e., higher prices for industrialized countries, lower prices for developing countries) (Berkley, in press), or the tax credits proposed by The Lifesaving Vaccine Technology Act of 1999 (U.S. House of Representatives, 1999). Further, it is necessary to create a policy environment that will assure the production and distribution of appropriate products when they are developed (Berkley, in press).

Of course, should a suitable vaccine or microbicide candidate be developed, certain pragmatic and ethical issues will need to be taken into consideration. For example, it will be important to have a comprehensive public relations and education plan in place that can help to balance the optimism surrounding the new product with realistic estimates of risks, resources, and the time needed to determine its protective efficacy (Langan and Collins, 1998). Additionally, it will be necessary to ensure that mechanisms are in place to protect the rights and health of clinical trial participants. Further, should a vaccine or microbicide candidate be proven safe and effective, there should be mechanisms in place to ensure broad public access to the new product (Langan and Collins, 1998). Resolving these issues will require the collaborative efforts of the Department of Health and Human Services and other federal agencies, state and local organizations, and advocacy groups. But despite such challenges, the promise of technological advances remains bright.

Therefore, the Committee recommends:

Federal agencies should continue to invest in the development of products and technologies linked to HIV prevention. In particular, the National Institutes of Health should place high priority on the development of anti-HIV microbicides and vaccines, and this prioritization should be accompanied by increases in funding. Similarly, the Food and Drug Administration should accelerate its efforts to approve prevention technologies that show promise in clinical trials (e.g., new antiretroviral therapies, new microbicidal and vaccine candidates) or are already being successfully utilized elsewhere in the world (e.g., rapid testing assays other than the Single Use Diagnostic System [SUDS]). For all new prevention tools, investigations of cost-effectiveness and user acceptability should be included as part of the research agenda. Federal agencies should also seek to develop stronger research collaborations with private industry, and they should offer incentives to encourage private industry investment.

REFERENCES

Anderson JE, Carey JW, Taveras S. 2000. HIV testing among the general US population and persons at increased risk: Information from national surveys, 1987–1996. *American Journal of Public Health* 90(7):1089–1095.

Andersson S, da Silva Z, Norrgren H, Dias F, Biberfeld G. 1997. Field evaluation of alternative testing strategies for diagnosis and differentiation of HIV-1 and HIV-2 infections in an HIV-1 and HIV-2-prevalent area. *AIDS* 11(15):1815–1822.

Bayer R, Stryker J, Smith MD. 1995. Testing for HIV infection at home. *New England Journal of Medicine* 1995 332(19):1296–1299.

Berkley S. In press. International Perspectives on HIV Vaccine Development. In Wong-Stall F and Gallo R (eds.), *AIDS Vaccine Research in Perspective*. New York: Marcel Dekker Inc.

Berman PW, Gray AM, Wrin T, Vennari JC, Eastman DJ, Nakamura GR, Francis DP, Gorse G, Schwartz DH. 1997. Genetic and immunologic characterization of viruses infecting MN-rgp120-vaccinated volunteers. *Journal of Infectious Diseases* 176(2):384–397.

Bird KD. 1991. The use of spermicide containing nonoxynol-9 in the prevention of HIV infection. *AIDS* 5(7):791–796.

Blakeslee DJ. 2000. Microbicides and pharm policy. [Web Page]. Located at: www.ama-assn.org/special/hiv/newsline/conferen/microb00/dbpharm.htm. Accessed June 7, 2000.

Blower SM, McLean AR. 1994. Prophylactic vaccines, risk behavior change, and the probability of eradicating HIV in San Francisco. *Science* 265(5177):1451–1454.

Centers for Disease Control and Prevention (CDC). 1996. HIV Counseling and Testing in Publicly Funded Sites: 1996 Annual Report. Atlanta: CDC.

Centers for Disease Control and Prevention (CDC). 1998. Update: HIV counseling and testing using rapid tests—United States, 1995. *Morbidity and Mortality Weekly Report* 47(11):211–215.

Centers for Disease Control and Prevention (CDC). 2000a. Notice to Readers: CDC statement on study results of product containing nonoxynol-9. *Morbidity and Mortality Weekly Report* 49(31):717.

Centers for Disease Control and Prevention (CDC). 2000b. A sero-status approach to fighting the HIV/AIDS epidemic. Atlanta, Georgia.

Collier AC, Coombs RW, Schoenfeld DA, Bassett RL, Timpone J, Baruch A, Jones M, Facey K, Whitacre C, McAuliffe VJ, Friedman HM, Merigan TC, Reichman RC, Hooper C, Corey L. 1996. Treatment of human immunodeficiency virus infection with saquinavir, zidovudine, and zalcitabine. AIDS Clinical Trials Group. *New England Journal of Medicine* 334(16):1011–1017.

Connor EM, Sperling RS, Gelber R, Kiselev P, Scott G, O'Sullivan MJ, VanDyke R, Bey M, Shearer W, Jacobson RL, Jimenez E, O'Neill E, Bazin B, Delfraissy JF, Culnane M, Coombs R, Elkins M, Moye J, Stratton P, Balsley J. 1994. Reduction of maternal–infant transmission of human immunodeficiency virus type 1 with zidovudine treatment. Pediatric AIDS Clinical Trials Group Protocol 076 Study Group. *New England Journal of Medicine* 331(18):1173–1180.

d'Oro LC, Parazzini F, Naldi L, La Vecchia C. 1994. Barrier methods of contraception, spermicides, and sexually transmitted diseases: a review. *Genitourinary Medicine* 70(6):410–417.

Davis KR and Weller SC. 1999. The effectiveness of condoms in reducing heterosexual transmission of HIV. *Family Planning Perspectives* 31(6):272–279.

de Zoysa I, Elias CJ, Bentley ME. 1998. Ethical challenges in efficacy trials of vaginal microbicides for HIV prevention. *American Journal of Public Health* 88(4):571–575.

Deeks SG, Smith M, Holodniy M, Kahn JO. 1997. HIV-1 protease inhibitors. A review for clinicians. *Journal of the American Medical Association* 277(2):145–153.

Dilley JW, Woods WJ, McFarland W. 1997. Are advances in treatment changing views about high-risk sex? *New England Journal of Medicine* 337(7):501–502.

El-Bassel N, Krishnan SP, Schilling RF, Witte S, Gilbert L. 1998. Acceptability of the female condom among STD clinic patients. *AIDS Education and Prevention* 10(5):465–480.

Elias CJ and Coggins C. 1996. Female-controlled methods to prevent sexual transmission of HIV. *AIDS* 10 (Suppl 3):S43–S51.

Farr G, Gabelnick H, Sturgen K, Dorflinger L. 1994. Contraceptive efficacy and acceptability of the female condom. *American Journal of Public Health* 84(12):1960–1964.

Feldblum PJ, Morrison CS, Roddy RE, Cates W Jr. 1995. The effectiveness of barrier methods of contraception in preventing the spread of HIV. *AIDS* 9 (Suppl A):S85–S93.

Forbes A. 1997 Beyond Male Condoms: Demanding a Woman-Controlled Prevention Tool [Web Page]. Located at: hivinsite.uscf.edu/topics/women/2098.355c.html.

Gibson S, McFarland W, Wohlfeiler D, Scheer K, Katz MH. 1999. Experiences of 100 men who have sex with men using the Reality condom for anal sex. *AIDS Education and Prevention* 11(1):65–71.

Global Forum for Health Research. 1999. The 10/90 Report on Health Research. Geneva, Switzerland: Global Forum for Health Research.

Grobman WA and Garcia PM. 1999. The cost-effectiveness of voluntary intrapartum rapid human immunodeficiency virus testing for women without adequate prenatal care. *American Journal of Obstetrics and Gynecology* 181(5 Pt 1):1062–1071.

Gulick RM, Mellors JW, Havlir D, Eron JJ, Gonzalez C, McMahon D, Richman DD, Valentine FT, Jonas L, Meibohm A, Emini EA, Chodakewitz JA, Deutsch P, Holder S, Schleif WA, Condra JH. 1997. Treatment with indinavir, zidovudine, and lamivudine in adults with human immunodeficiency virus infection and prior antiretroviral therapy. *New England Journal of Medicine* 337(11):734–739.

Heise L. 2000. Presentation. Microbicides 2000; Mar 13–16, 2000 Mar 16; Alexandria, Virginia.

Institute of Medicine. 1999. *Reducing the Odds: Preventing Perinatal Transmission of HIV in the United States.* Stoto MA, Almario DA, and McCormick MC (Eds.). Washington, DC: National Academy Press.

International AIDS Vaccine Initiative (IAVI). 2000. Public policy initiatives to accelerate the global search for an effective AIDS vaccine. [Web Page] Located at: www.iavi.org/globalmobil_z_ economics_3-4-1.html.

International Working Group on Vaginal Microbicides. 1996. Recommendations for the development of vaginal microbicides. *AIDS* 10(8):1–6.

Irwin K, Olivo N, Schable CA, Weber JT, Janssen R, Ernst J. 1996. Performance characteristics of a rapid HIV antibody assay in a hospital with a high prevalence of HIV infection. CDC-Bronx-Lebanon HIV Serosurvey Team. *Annals of Internal Medicine* 125(6):471–475.

Joint United Nations Programme on HIV/AIDS. 2000. "Greater Private Sector Involvement needed in Microbicide Research, Says UNAIDS Chief." Press Release, March.

Kalichman SC, Nachimson D, Cherry C, Williams E. 1998. AIDS treatment advances and behavioral prevention setbacks: Preliminary assessment of reduced perceived threat of HIV-AIDS. *Health Psychology* 17(6):546–550.

Kamb ML, Fishbein M, Douglas JM Jr, Rhodes F, Rogers J, Bolan G, Zenilman J, Hoxworth T, Malotte CK, Iatesta M, Kent, Lentz A, Graziano S, Byers RH, Peterman TA. 1998. Efficacy of risk-reduction counseling to prevent human immunodeficiency virus and sexually transmitted diseases: a randomized controlled trial. Project RESPECT Study Group. *Journal of the American Medical Association* 280(13):1161–1167.

Kane B. 1999. Rapid testing for HIV: Why so fast? *Annals of Internal Medicine* 131(6):481–483.

Kassler WJ. 1997. Advances in HIV testing technology and their potential impact on prevention. *AIDS Education and Prevention* 9(3 Suppl):27–40.

Kassler WJ, Dillon BA, Haley C, Jones WK, Goldman A. 1997. On-site, rapid HIV testing with same-day results and counseling. *AIDS* 11(8):1045–1051.

Kassler WJ, Haley C, Jones WK, Gerber AR, Kennedy EJ, George JR. 1995. Performance of a rapid, on-site human immunodeficiency virus antibody assay in a public health setting. *Journal of Clinical Microbiology* 33(11):2899–2902.

Kelen GD, Hexter DA, Hansen KN, Tang N, Pretorius S, Quinn TC. 1995. Trends in human immunodeficiency virus (HIV) infection among a patient population of an inner-city emergency department: implications for emergency department-based screening programs for HIV infection. *Clinical Infectious Diseases* 21(4):867–875.

Kelen GD, Shahan JB, Quinn TC. 1999. Emergency department-based HIV screening and counseling: Experience with rapid and standard serologic testing. *Annals of Emergency Medicine* 33(2):147–155.

Kelly JA, Hoffman RG, Rompa D, Gray M. 1998a. Protease inhibitor combination therapies and perceptions of gay men regarding AIDS severity and the need to maintain safer sex. *AIDS* 12(10):F91–F95.

Kelly JA, Otto-Salaj LL, Sikkema KJ, Pinkerton SD, Bloom FR. 1998b. Implications of HIV treatment advances for behavioral research on AIDS: Protease inhibitors and new challenges in HIV secondary prevention. *Health Psychology* 17(4):310–319.

Kimball AM, Berkley S, Ngugi E, Gayle H. 1995. International aspects of the AIDS/HIV epidemic. *Annual Review of Public Health* 16:253–282.

Klein H, Eber M, Crosby H, Welka DA, Hoffman JA. 1999. The acceptability of the female condom among substance-using women in Washington, DC. *Women's Health* 29(3):97–114.

Kravcik S, Victor G, Houston S, Sutherland D, Garber GE, Hawley-Foss N, Angel JB, Cameron DW. 1998. Effect of antiretroviral therapy and viral load on the perceived risk of HIV transmission and the need for safer sexual practices. *Journal of Acquired Immune Deficiency Syndromes and Human and Retrovirology* 19(2):124–129.

Kremer M. 2000a. Creating markets for new vaccines, part I: Rationale. Cambridge, MA: National Bureau of Economic Research, Working Paper 7716.

Kremer M. 2000b. Creating markets for new vaccines, part II: Design Issues. Cambridge, MA: National Bureau of Economic Research, Working Paper 7717.

Langan M and Collins C. 1998. Paving the road to an HIV vaccine: Employing tools of public policy to overcome scientific, economic, social, and ethical obstacles. University of California, AIDS Research Institute Monograph.

Lawson L, Katzenstein D, Vermund S. 1999. Emerging Biomedical Interventions. In Gibney L, DiClimente RJ, and Vermund SH, (Eds.), *Preventing HIV in Developing Countries*: Biomedical and Behavioral Approaches. New York: Kluwer Academic/Plenum Publishers.

Lindsay MK, Grant J, Peterson HB, Risby J, Williams H, Klein L. 1993. Human immunodeficiency virus infection among patients in a gynecology emergency department. *Obstetrics and Gynecology* 81(6):1012–1015.

Madrigal J, Schifter J, Feldblum PJ. 1998. Female condom acceptability among sex workers in Costa Rica. *AIDS Education and Prevention* 10(2):105–113.

Malkovsky M, Newell A, Dalgleish AG. 1988. Inactivation of HIV by nonoxynol-9. *Lancet* 1(8586):645.

McGill W, Miller K, Bolan G, Malotte K, Zenilman J, Iatesta M, Kamb M, Douglas J. 1998. Awareness of and experience with the female condom among patients attending STD clinics. *Sexually Transmitted Diseases* 25(4):222–223.

Meda N, Gautier-Charpentier L, Soudre RB, Dahourou H, Ouedraogo-Traore R, Ouangre A, Bambara A, Kpozehouen A, Sanou H, Valea D, Ky F, Cartoux M, Barin F, Van de Perre P. 1999. Serological diagnosis of human immuno-deficiency virus in Burkina Faso: Reliable, practical strategies using less expensive commercial test kits. *Bulletin of the World Health Organization* 77(9):731–739.

Miller CJ, Gerstein MJ, Davis RC, Katz DH. 1995. N-docosanol prevents vaginal transmission of SIVmac251 in rhesus macaques (Abstract 97). Eighth International Conference on Antiviral Research; Apr 23–Apr 28, 1995; Santa Fe, New Mexico.

Mitchell D. 2000 Mar 15. Vaginal microbicide conference highlights HIV prevention. Reuters Health Information.

Musaba E, Morrison CS, Sunkutu MR, Wong EL. 1998. Long-term use of the female condom among couples at high risk of human immunodeficiency virus infection in Zambia. *Sexually Transmitted Diseases* 25(5):260–264.

Musicco M, Lazzarin A, Nicolosi A, Gasparini M, Costigliola P, Arici C, Saracco A. 1994. Antiretroviral treatment of men infected with human immunodeficiency virus type 1 reduces the incidence of heterosexual transmission. Italian Study Group on HIV Heterosexual Transmission. *Archives of Internal Medicine* 154(17):1971–1976.

Neurath AR, Jiang S, Strick N, Lin K, Li YY, Debnath AK. 1996. Bovine beta-lactoglobulin modified by 3-hydroxyphthalic anhydride blocks the CD4 cell receptor for HIV. *Nature Medicine* 2(2):230–234.

Pearce-Pratt R. and Phillips DM. 1996. Sulfated polysaccharides inhibit lymphocyte-to-epithelial transmission of human immunodeficiency virus-1. *Biology of Reproduction* 54(1):173–182.

Pinkerton SD and Abramson PR. 1997. Effectiveness of condoms in preventing HIV transmission. *Social Science and Medicine* 44(9):1303–1312.

Population Council and International Family Health. 2000. *The Case for Microbicides: A Global Priority.* New York: Population Council and International Family Health.

Quinn TC, Wawer MJ, Sewankambo N, Serwadda D, Li C, Wabwire-Mangen F, Meehan MO, Lutalo T, Gray RH. 2000. Viral load and heterosexual transmission of human immunodeficiency virus type 1. Rakai Project Study Group. *New England Journal of Medicine* 342(13):921–929.

Ragni MV, Faruki H, Kingsley LA. 1998. Heterosexual HIV-1 transmission and viral load in hemophilic patients. *Journal of Acquired Immune Deficiency Syndromes and Human and Retrovirology* 17(1):42–45.

Redondo-Lopez V, Cook RL, Sobel JD. 1990. Emerging role of lactobacilli in the control and maintenance of the vaginal bacterial microflora. *Review of Infectious Diseases* 12(5):856–872.

Roddy RE, Schulz KF, Cates W Jr. 1998a. Microbicides, meta-analysis, and the N-9 question. Where's the research? *Sexually Transmitted Diseases* 25(3):151–153.

Roddy RE, Zekeng L, Ryan KA, Tamoufe U, Weir SS, Wong EL. 1998b. A controlled trial of nonoxynol 9 film to reduce male-to-female transmission of sexually transmitted diseases. *New England Journal of Medicine* 339(8):504–510.

Rotheram-Borus MJ, Gillis JR, Reid HM, Fernandez MI, Gwadz M. 1997. HIV testing, behaviors, and knowledge among adolescents at high risk. *Journal of Adolescent Health* 20(3):216–225.

Royce RA, Sena A, Cates W Jr, Cohen MS. 1997. Sexual transmission of HIV. *New England Journal of Medicine* 336(15):1072–1078.

Schwartz DH, Gorse G, Clements ML, Belshe R, Izu A, Duliege AM, Berman P, Twaddell T, Stablein D, Sposto R, Siliciano R, Matthews T. 1993. Induction of HIV-1-neutralising and syncytium-inhibiting antibodies in uninfected recipients of HIV-1IIIB rgp120 subunit vaccine. *Lancet* 342(8863):69–73.

Seal DW, Ehrhardt AA. 1999. Heterosexual men's attitudes toward the female condom. *AIDS Education and Prevention* 11(2):93–106.

Shervington DO. 1993. The acceptability of the female condom among low-income African-American women. *Journal of the National Medical Association* 85(5):341–347.

Solomon L, Stein M, Flynn C, Schuman P, Schoenbaum E, Moore J, Holmberg S, Graham NM. 1998. Health services use by urban women with or at risk for HIV-1 infection: The HIV Epidemiology Research Study (HERS). *Journal of Acquired Immune Deficiency Syndromes and Human and Retrovirology* 17(3):253–261.

Soper DE, Shoupe D, Shangold GA, Shangold MM, Gutmann J, Mercer L. 1993. Prevention of vaginal trichomoniasis by compliant use of the female condom. *Sexually Transmitted Diseases* 20(3):137–139.

Stephenson J. 2000. AIDS researchers explore new drug options. *Journal of the American Medical Association* 283(9):1125.

Stetler HC, Granade TC, Nunez CA, Meza R, Terrell S, Amador L, George JR. 1997. Field evaluation of rapid HIV serologic tests for screening and confirming HIV-1 infection in Honduras. *AIDS* 11(3):369–375.

Thompson KA, Malamud D, Storey BT. 1996. Assessment of the anti-microbial agent C31G as a spermicide: Comparison with nonoxynol-9. *Contraception* 53(5):313–318.

Trussell J, Sturgen K, Strickler J, Dominik R. 1994. Comparative contraceptive efficacy of the female condom and other barrier methods. *Family Planning Perspective* 26(2):66–72.

U.S. House of Representatives. 1999. Lifesaving vaccine technology act of 1999. 106th Congress, 1st Session, House of Representatives.

Valdiserri RO, Moore M, Gerber AR, Campbell CH Jr, Dillon BA, West GR. 1993. A study of clients returning for counseling after HIV testing: Implications for improving rates of return. *Public Health Reports* 108(1):12–18.

Van Damme L. 2000. Advances in topical microbicides (Session P104). XIII International AIDS Conference; Jul 9–Jul 14, 2000; Durban, South Africa.

Van Damme L, and Rosenberg Z. 1999. Microbicides and barrier methods in HIV prevention. *AIDS* 13(Suppl):S85–S92.

Vanable PA, Ostrow DG, McKirnan DJ, Taywaditep KJ, Hope BA. 2000. Impact of combination therapies on HIV risk perceptions and sexual risk among HIV-positive and HIV-negative gay and bisexual men. *Health Psychology* 19(2):134–145.

Vanchieri C. 1996. Experts plan for next generation of HIV tests. *Annals of Internal Medicine* 125(6):162–63.

Voeller B and Anderson DJ. 1992. Vaginal pH and related factors in the urogenital tract and rectum that affect HIV-1 transmission (Mariposa Occasional Paper No. 16). Topanga, CA: The Mariposa Education and Research Foundation.

The Voluntary HIV-1 Counseling and Testing Efficacy Study Group. 2000. Efficacy of voluntary HIV-1 counselling and testing in individuals and couples in Kenya, Tanzania, and Trinidad: A randomised trial. *Lancet* 356(9224):103–112.

Weinhardt LS, Carey MP, Johnson BT, Bickham NL. 1999. Effects of HIV counseling and testing on sexual risk behavior: A meta-analytic review of published research, 1985–1997. *American Journal of Public Health* 89(9):1397–1405.

Weller SC. 1993. A meta-analysis of condom effectiveness in reducing sexually transmitted HIV. *Social Science and Medicine* 36(12):1635–1644.

Witte SS, El-Bassel N, Wada T, Gray O, Wallace J. 1999. Acceptability of female condom use among women exchanging street sex in New York City. *International Journal of STDs and AIDS* 10(3):162–168.

Wulf D, Frost J, Darroch JE. 1999. *Microbicides: A New Defense against Sexually Transmitted Diseases.* Washington, DC: Alan Guttmacher Institute.

7

Overcoming Social Barriers

Although major accomplishments have been made in HIV prevention over the past 20 years, a number of unrealized opportunities
to avert new infections still exist. These missed opportunities derive from underlying social and political barriers that have acted as constraints to the objective of preventing as many new infections as possible.
Among the most pernicious of the social barriers are poverty, racism,
gender inequality, AIDS-related stigma, and society's reluctance to openly
address sexuality. Other important barriers have been the lack of leadership by political and national leaders in galvanizing efforts to combat the
epidemic, as well as misperceptions about HIV/AIDS among many
people at risk for becoming infected. These barriers have had a profound
effect on the course of the HIV epidemic by influencing risk behaviors
and by promoting a social context in which HIV transmission is likely to
occur. The barriers also have had a fundamental bearing on public policy
decisions regarding funding, research, and treatment, and they have influenced decisions about which prevention programs are implemented,
the mechanisms by which they occur, and the populations targeted.

The Committee believes that while these entrenched barriers cannot
be easily overcome, they must nevertheless be explicitly acknowledged in
HIV prevention efforts. The Committee also believes that specific policies
and laws emanating from these social and political conditions and attitudes can and must be changed. In this chapter, we describe the barriers
that influence the epidemic, and we identify four specific instances in

which these conditions and attitudes have resulted in public policies that run counter to scientific knowledge about effective HIV prevention.

SOCIAL BARRIERS

Poverty, Racism, and Gender Inequality

There is considerable evidence that social inequalities defined by income, race, ethnicity, and gender are key elements in the social contexts and environments that contribute to HIV infection risk. These contextual forces can act at the individual level, when life circumstances such as homelessness or drug use increase the likelihood of high-risk behaviors. The forces also can act at the societal level (Henderson, 1988). For example, economic inequalities between women and men can affect women's perceptions of their ability to negotiate safe sex practices in a social relationship. Similarly, racism—both historically and in its contemporary forms—has resulted in assaults on the economic opportunities and the self-identity of racial and ethnic minorities, and has implications for Americans' receptivity to HIV prevention efforts. Moreover, social inequalities create conditions that make it difficult for individuals and communities to even focus on the problem of HIV, since other problems may seem more immediate (e.g., housing, employment). Better understanding these societal forces is critical to achieving the objective of preventing as many new infections as possible.

Increasingly, the metropolitan areas that are most severely affected by HIV/AIDS are also areas of social and political neglect. Individuals living in these disenfranchised environments have increased exposure to a variety of social and psychosocial factors (e.g., poverty, stress, disrupted family structures, insufficient social supports, and toxic environmental exposures) that have demonstrated associations with morbidity and mortality (Geronimus, 2000). Further, inadequate access to health care and lack of supportive, culturally appropriate social services allow co-occurring conditions—such as substance abuse, mental illness, tuberculosis, sexually transmitted diseases (STDs), and violence—to flourish, thus forming epidemiological clusters for a wide variety of concurrent health and social problems (NRC, 1993). Moreover, the higher prevalence of drug trade in impoverished neighborhoods increases the likelihood of exposure to and use of drugs, such as heroin, crack, and cocaine, that are linked to HIV risk (Zierler and Krieger, 1997). These findings are consistent with studies documenting the correlation between economic deprivation and overall AIDS incidence at the state level (Zierler et al., 2000) and in major metropolitan areas (Fordyce et al., 1998; Simon et al., 1995; Hu et al., 1994; Fife and Mode, 1992).

Given that racial and ethnic minority groups are also over-represented among those with HIV/AIDS (see Appendix A; CDC, 2000a), the added burden of coping with societal racism further complicates the implementation of HIV prevention efforts, especially in urban communities. In many urban areas, a legacy of discriminatory social policies (e.g., racially biased mortgage practices, siting of public housing projects and transportation routes) has resulted in a concentration of racial and ethnic minorities in neighborhoods isolated from the social and health care infrastructures needed to preserve health (Cohen and Northridge, 2000; Gerominus, 2000). In addition, racism in the health care setting can pose a major barrier to engaging members of racial and ethnic minority groups in care and prevention efforts (Bayne-Smith, 1996). In one survey of racial and ethnic minorities, 98 percent of respondents reported experiencing some type of racial discrimination within the past year, and 55 percent reported discrimination by health care professionals (Landrine and Klonoff, 1997). Historical accounts of racism in the medical establishment (e.g., the Tuskegee Syphilis Study) have fostered a lack of trust in the modern health care system among some minority groups (Thomas and Quinn, 1991). For example, a recent survey found that 27 percent of African-American respondents believed that HIV/AIDS is a government conspiracy against their racial group (Klonoff and Landrine, 1999). The distrust and fear derived from racist experiences and historical traumas have serious implications for carrying out effective HIV prevention and treatment activities in minority communities. If prevention efforts are to succeed in reaching racial and ethnic minorities, then they must take into account the impact of racism and explicitly address these types of concerns in developing scientifically sound, ethnically appropriate, and culturally acceptable interventions (Thomas and Quinn, 1991).

Over the past two decades, women have represented a steadily increasing proportion of AIDS cases (see Appendix A; CDC, 2000a). Because a substantial and increasing proportion of women are infected through heterosexual contact, HIV prevention strategies broadly targeted to women have stressed women's negotiation skills in sexual decision making as a way to change male behavior, rather than targeting male behavior directly. This strategy assumes, however, that women have control in sexual decision making and that relations between the genders are equal, which is often not true (Campbell, 1995).

In many cases, gender inequality and the consequences that can derive from it (e.g., domestic violence, fear of abandonment) contribute to a social environment in which a woman may be either unable or unwilling to negotiate consistent condom use or lower-risk sexual practices (Zierler and Krieger, 1997). In extreme instances, initiating discussions of condom use and risk reduction may lead to physical or sexual abuse (Lurie et al.,

1995). Gender inequality may be extreme for drug-addicted women and for those whose partners use drugs, as a large proportion of these women report histories of childhood or adult sexual abuse (Walker et al., 1992; Cohen et al., 2000). In fact, there is a growing body of evidence linking childhood or adolescent sexual abuse to behavioral sequelae that increase risk for HIV infection in adulthood (Zierler and Krieger, 1997). In addition, for some women, sexual risk behavior may be tied to practices (e.g., commercial sex work) that ensure economic survival for themselves and their families. For these reasons, it is essential to acknowledge that gender inequality affects many women and must be taken into account when creating prevention messages for women.

The Sexual "Code of Silence"

Society's reluctance to openly confront issues regarding sexuality results in a number of untoward effects. This social inhibition impedes the development and implementation of effective sexual health and HIV/STD education programs, and it stands in the way of communication between parents and children and between sex partners (IOM, 1997b). It perpetuates misperceptions about individual risk and ignorance about the consequences of sexual activities and may encourage high-risk sexual practices (Gerrard, 1982, 1987). It also impacts the level of counseling training given to health care providers to assess sexual histories, as well as providers' comfort levels in conducting risk-behavior discussions with clients (ARHP and ANPRH, 1995; Risen, 1995; Makadon and Silin, 1995; Merrill et al., 1990). In addition, the "code of silence" has resulted in missed opportunities to use the mass media (e.g., television, radio, printed media, and the Internet) to encourage healthy sexual behaviors (IOM, 1997b; NRC, 1989). The media can be powerful allies in promoting knowledge about HIV and other STDs, and in fostering behavioral change that can reduce the chances of acquiring these diseases (STD Communication Roundtable, 1996). For example, while both children and adolescents are constantly exposed to—and particularly vulnerable to—explicit and implicit sexual messages in various media, the presence of prevention messages (e.g., use of condoms) in the media is practically nonexistent (Lowry and Shidler, 1993; Harris and Associates, 1988). Further, because many adolescents are not receiving accurate information regarding drugs, STDs, and healthy sexual behavior from their parents or other trusted adult sources, they often rely on the media as a primary source of information (STD Communication Roundtable, 1996). Given the impact of media on young people's attitudes, as well as on consumer behavior, messages that consistently promote risk reduction could facilitate much-needed changes in social norms regarding sexual behaviors and drug-use practices.

TEXT BOX 7.1
Recommendations from *The Hidden Epidemic*

The Hidden Epidemic made two major recommendations in terms of developing a new social norm of sexual behavior as the basis for long-term prevention of STDs. These recommendations are:

1. An independent, long-term national campaign should be established to: (a) serve as a catalyst for social change toward a new norm of healthy sexual behavior in the United States; (b) support and implement a long-term national initiative to increase knowledge and awareness of STDs and promote ways to prevent them; and (c) develop a standing committee to function as an expert resource and to develop guidelines and resources for incorporating messages regarding STDs and healthy sexual behaviors into all forms of mass media.

2. Television, radio, print, music, and other mass media companies should accept advertisements and sponsor public service messages that promote condom use and other means of protecting against STDs and unintended pregnancy, including delaying sexual intercourse.

In order to address the public's reluctance to openly confront and discuss sexuality and sexual health, the Committee wishes to acknowledge and endorse recommendations from a prior Institute of Medicine report, *The Hidden Epidemic*, which aimed to catalyze social change by encouraging discussion of these issues and by promoting balanced mass media messages (IOM, 1997b). Specifically, the report called for a significant national campaign to foster social change that would lead to a new norm of healthy sexual behavior. This campaign would make extensive use of the media to promote comprehensive public health messages regarding STDs, HIV infection, sexual abuse, and unintended pregnancy (Text Box 7.1). The strategies set forth in *The Hidden Epidemic* recommendations, if they were implemented, would constitute significant steps toward changing social and cultural norms and beliefs about sex.

Stigma of HIV/AIDS

Since the beginning of the HIV/AIDS epidemic, people living with HIV or AIDS have been the targets of stigma and discrimination. Despite two decades of public education, prevention efforts, and passage of protective legislation, AIDS-related stigma continues to be a serious problem (Herek, 1999). AIDS stigma is manifested through discrimination and social ostracism directed against individuals with HIV or AIDS, against groups of people perceived to be likely to be infected, and against those individuals, groups, and communities with whom these individuals interact (Herek and Capitanio, 1998).

AIDS stigma is closely linked to other existing social prejudices, including prejudice against homosexuals and drug users. The initial identification of HIV/AIDS among these marginalized groups has had a lasting impact on the way in which the disease is perceived by the American public. Throughout the 1980s, many people closely associated the AIDS epidemic with homosexual behavior and, although the epidemiology of HIV/AIDS has changed considerably, most heterosexual adults continue to associate AIDS with homosexuality or bisexuality (Herek and Capitanio, 1999). In a 1997 survey, 45 percent of respondents thought that a healthy man could get AIDS by having sex with another *uninfected* man (Herek and Capitanio, 1999). The public also assigns more blame to people who contract HIV/AIDS through behavior that is perceived as controllable (e.g., sex, sharing needles). In the same 1997 survey, 98 percent of respondents felt sympathy for a person who contracted AIDS through a blood transfusion, while only 58 percent felt sympathy for someone who has contracted the virus through homosexual contact (Herek and Capitanio, 1999). Similarly, AIDS-related stigma has combined with stigma of drug use to affect public policy about HIV prevention programs that target injection drug users (IDUs). For instance, there continues to be strong opposition to needle exchange programs, despite strong evidence of their efficacy (Herek et al., 1998).

In the United States, a significant minority of the public has expressed consistently negative attitudes toward persons living with AIDS and has supported blatantly stigmatizing and punitive measures against them (Herek, 1999). Such actions have helped foster widespread public stigma toward those who are HIV-infected or even perceived to have AIDS, resulting in overt discriminatory practices (such as denial of housing or employment), violence, social prejudice, and moral judgments (Herek and Glunt, 1988; Herek and Capitanio, 1998). Fortunately, support for such measures has declined over time. A national survey conducted in 1991 found that 36 percent of the population supported quarantines for HIV-infected persons and 30 percent supported public disclosure of the names of infected persons; the same survey conducted in 1997 found that these percentages had dropped to 17 percent and 19 percent, respectively (Herek and Capitanio, 1998). Further, the 1997 survey indicated that the majority (77 percent) of respondents believed that people with AIDS are unfairly persecuted in our society (Herek and Capitanio, 1998).

However, there are disturbing trends, too. Compared to 1991, more respondents agreed that people who acquired AIDS through sex or drug use got what they deserved (29 percent in 1997 versus 20 percent in 1991). Similarly, the proportion of the public that believes casual social contact might lead to HIV infection has increased somewhat (Herek and Capitanio, 1998). In 1991, 55 percent of respondents believed it was possible to contract AIDS from using the same drinking glass (compared with 48 percent in 1991), and 54 percent believed that AIDS might be transmitted through a cough or sneeze (compared to 45 percent in 1991).

AIDS stigma has serious implications for carrying out effective prevention efforts. At-risk or HIV-infected individuals who fear stigmatization or being labeled as part of a stigmatized social group may be reluctant to admit risk behaviors, to seek or find relevance in prevention information, to obtain antibody testing, or to access health care services (Chesney and Smith, 1999; Herek, 1999). These factors can increase the likelihood of continuing risk behaviors, becoming infected, and transmitting the virus to others (Herek et al., 1998).

Thus, while some progress has been made in reducing AIDS stigma, and while public support for discriminatory policies has diminished, AIDS stigma still persists and continues to undermine HIV prevention efforts. As a result, the Committee believes that the protection of human rights, privacy, and equity continues to be a significant concern, and that concurrent efforts at the federal, state, and local level to remove or at least lessen the impact of stigma and discrimination are necessary. In this belief, the Committee states its unflinching commitment to the protection of the rights of those living with HIV/AIDS and those at risk for HIV.

Misperceptions

In addition to the social conditions and attitudes that impede HIV prevention efforts, many people at risk for becoming infected have a variety of misperceptions about HIV/AIDS that hinder the effectiveness of prevention efforts. Several studies have shown that individuals often underestimate or misperceive their risk of acquiring HIV (Mays and Cochran, 1988; Schieman, 1998; Kaiser Family Foundation, 1999a) and STDs (IOM, 1997b), which can lead to an increase in risk behaviors. This misperception is driven, in large part, by the complexity of exposure to HIV: the uncertainty of exposure, the low probability of infection per encounter, the time interval between infection and clinical manifestation of HIV, and the emotional reaction to the severity of AIDS (Poppen and Reisen, 1997). Studies have shown that general knowledge about HIV does not necessarily predict practice of preventive behaviors (Mickler, 1993). Even when individuals are worried about contracting HIV, their perception of the likelihood of actually contracting HIV often is relatively low (Dolcini et al., 1996; Ford and Norris, 1993). Individuals who do not consider themselves to be in "high-risk groups" perceive themselves at low risk and thus engage in riskier behaviors (Dolcini et al., 1996; Mickler,

1993; Lewis et al., 1997). Another belief that influences individuals' risk behavior is their misperception about HIV-infected people. For example, some individuals believe that anyone who "looks healthy" must not have AIDS, which may lead these individuals to be falsely confident in selecting partners (Ford and Norris, 1993). Finally, the stigma associated with HIV/AIDS can affect the perception of high-risk behavior. People who engage in high-risk activities believed to be behaviorally irresponsible, such as injecting drugs or having unprotected sex, may dissociate from their own behaviors and rationalize that they are not at risk for contracting HIV (Poppen and Reisen, 1997).

The success of combination antiretroviral therapies, along with the emphasis on vaccine development, has also led some people to believe that they no longer need to take precautions against transmitting or acquiring HIV. For example, in a study of HIV-negative or untested persons at risk, 17 percent reported that they were less careful about sex and drug use, and 31 percent were less concerned about becoming infected, because of new treatments (Lehman et al., 2000). In addition, recent studies indicate that treatment advances may have contributed to a resurgence in high-risk behaviors, particularly unprotected sex, as demonstrated by the increased incidence of STDs in San Francisco (CDC, 1999a), Seattle (CDC, 1999b; Williams et al., 1999), Los Angeles, and Philadelphia (Marquis, 2000), particularly among men who have sex with men.

Lack of Leadership

Concerted efforts by politicians and national leaders to openly discuss HIV and engage the public in HIV prevention efforts can set the stage for a national-level mobilization against the epidemic. The Committee believes that such high-level political commitment is necessary for developing a coherent strategy for responding to the epidemic and for providing leadership and direction to other public and private partners, such as federal, state, and local government agencies, community-based organizations, advocacy organizations, researchers, health care providers, the media, and affected communities. While several studies have made recommendations to resolve the interagency[1] and intraagency[2] co-

---

[1]The 1994 report to Philip Lee, then Assistant Secretary of Health, made strong recommendations aimed at resolving many of the coordination and leadership issues within the Department of Health and Human Services (DHHS, 1994).

[2]The 1999 review of the CDC's HIV/AIDS activities by the CDC Advisory Council on HIV Prevention identified opportunities for improved programmatic and budgetary coordination within the agency (CDC Advisory Committee, 1999).

ordination and leadership problems at the federal level, the nation still lacks the federal leadership and integration of prevention activities necessary to effectively address the epidemic (CDC Advisory Committee, 1999; PACHA, 2000).

Although there are difficulties in developing coordinated public and private-sector leadership for prevention, such leadership is not impossible. Studies in select developing and industrialized countries reveal the critical roles of consistent, visible political leadership and commitment, along with community mobilization, in slowing the epidemic. For example, in Uganda, a country ravaged by HIV/AIDS, government leaders openly acknowledged the epidemic and took active steps to prevent its spread by creating, in 1986, a National AIDS Control Programme. The program, which involves collaborations among community, government, and donor agencies, includes extensive prevention education campaigns to promote safer sexual behavior, STD prevention and treatment, condom distribution, HIV counseling and testing, and community mobilization to promote behavior change (UNAIDS, 1998; Abdool Karim et al., 1998). These efforts have contributed to high levels of awareness about HIV/ AIDS and declines in HIV incidence among some populations in Uganda (UNAIDS, 2000; UNAIDS, 1998). Political commitment and strong public health programs have also helped Thailand reduce HIV incidence among some of its populations (UNAIDS, 1998; Nelson et al., 1996), and they have helped Senegal maintain one of the lowest HIV incidence rates in Africa (UNAIDS, 1999). Among industrialized countries, government leaders in Australia and the Netherlands have worked with communities to develop policies that minimize the harm incurred by drug abuse and reduce stigmatization of drug users. These countries offer drug abuse treatment on demand; they also have rapidly expanded the availability of methadone maintenance, and they have successfully developed innovative methods for targeting drug users and slowing the HIV/AIDS epidemic among IDUs (Drucker et al., 1998). Perhaps the most impressive aspect of these successes is that, in some cases, such leadership has occurred in countries that have fewer educational, financial, biomedical, and social resources than does the United States.

While there have been prevention successes in the United States as a result of community mobilization, these have generally occurred on a more localized scale and often in the absence of high-level political leadership. For example, community mobilization in the gay community in the early and mid-1980s led to significant changes in sexual behavior and declines in HIV incidence among MSMs in major urban epicenters such as New York and San Francisco (Katz, 1997). These efforts preceded the development of any official public education programs (NRC and IOM, 1993).

UNREALIZED OPPORTUNITIES

The Committee identified four specific instances in which the social and political barriers described above have led to public policies that run counter to the scientific evidence regarding the effectiveness of HIV prevention interventions. These instances involve access to drug abuse treatment, access to sterile drug injection equipment, comprehensive sex education and condom availability in schools, and HIV prevention in correctional settings. These examples fall into two categories: (1) those in which policies impede implementation of effective HIV prevention efforts, and (2) those in which policies encourage funding for programs with no evidence of effectiveness. We believe that continuing to support such policies will result in unnecessary new HIV infections, lives lost, and wasted expenditures.

Access to Drug Abuse Treatment and Sterile Injection Equipment

Injection drug use is a major factor in the spread of HIV in the United States, accounting for 22 percent of new AIDS cases in 1999 (CDC, 2000a). Although the primary route of transmission among IDUs is through sharing of contaminated injection equipment, sexual partners and children of IDUs are also at high risk for infection (NRC and IOM, 1995). Non-injection drug use (e.g., use of alcohol, methamphetamines, crack cocaine, inhalants) also increases the likelihood of HIV infection and transmission through increasing high-risk sexual behaviors (IOM, 1997b).

Two of the most effective strategies for preventing HIV infection among IDUs include eliminating or reducing the frequency of drug use and associated risk behaviors through drug abuse treatment, and reducing the frequency of sharing injection equipment through expanded access to sterile injection equipment. However, legal, regulatory, and funding barriers prevent widespread implementation of these interventions.

Access to Drug Abuse Treatment

Drug abuse treatment can be provided in a variety of care settings (e.g., outpatient, residential, inpatient) using two primary types of interventions: pharmacotherapy or psychosocial/behavioral therapy. Pharmacotherapy, such as methadone maintenance treatment for opiate addiction, relies on medication to block the euphoria of the drug and the cravings and withdrawal symptoms associated with drug dependency. Psychosocial/behavioral therapies include skills training or a variety of counseling approaches. Some programs combine elements of the two approaches; for instance, many methadone maintenance programs also utilize some form of counseling or psychotherapy (GAO, 1998).

Studies conducted over three decades have demonstrated the effectiveness of drug abuse treatment in reducing drug use (NIH, 1997a; GAO, 1998; OTA, 1990). Methadone maintenance has been the most rigorously studied treatment modality, and it has been shown to be the most effective approach for treating opiate addiction, particularly when combined with counseling, education, and other psychosocial support services (NIH, 1997b; GAO, 1998).[3] Methadone maintenance also has been associated with other positive outcomes such as improved social functioning among those on maintenance and decreased crime rates (GAO, 1998; NIH, 1997b; IOM, 1995b). The recent nationwide Drug Abuse Treatment Outcome Study concluded that other common forms of drug abuse treatment (long-term residential, outpatient drug free, and short-term inpatient programs), in addition to methadone maintenance, are also effective in reducing drug use and in improving social functioning for a variety of drug-using populations[4] (Hubbard et al., 1997). There is less agreement, however, about the most appropriate treatment approach and setting combinations for non-opiate drug abusing populations (GAO, 1998; IOM, 1990).

In recent years, a number of studies have found that drug abuse treatment also reduces risk behaviors associated with HIV/AIDS. Methadone maintenance, which reduces injection and needle-related behaviors that place individuals at risk for HIV have shown particular success (Broome et al., 1999; Magura et al., 1998; Camacho et al., 1996; Longshore et al., 1993; Ball et al., 1988). For example, one study of opiate-addicted IDUs found a six-fold difference in HIV seroconversion rates between those in methadone treatment (seroconversion of 3.5 percent) and addicts who did not enter treatment (seroconversion rate of 22 percent) (Metzger et al., 1993). Drug abuse treatment reduces sex-related risk behaviors (Broome et al., 1999; Magura et al., 1998; Camacho et al., 1996), although this is not a traditional objective of drug treatment (Broome et al., 1999) and earlier findings have been inconsistent (Fisher and Fisher, 1992).

Despite the effectiveness of treatment, many people who could benefit from treatment do not receive it. The Office of National Drug Control Policy estimates that, of the approximately 5 million individuals with

---

[3]While many drug treatment programs include basic services such as HIV testing and counseling (D'Aunno et al., 1999), few programs offer other important medical and psychosocial services (Friedman et al., 2000). While large amounts of ancillary support services are not cost-effective, moderate amounts of support are better than minimal support levels (Kraft et al., 1997). The cost-effectiveness and proper targeting of ancillary services to improve HIV risk behavior are areas that warrant further research.

[4]Cocaine was the most common drug of abuse in these settings, followed by alcohol (Hubbard et al., 1997).

chronic, severe drug problems in the United States in 1998,[5] only 2.1 million (43 percent) received treatment (ONDCP, 2000c). During the same year, approximately 20 percent of the estimated 810,000 heroin addicts were in methadone treatment (ONDCP, 2000a).

Many factors contribute to this treatment gap, including insufficient public and private funding to provide treatment on request, restrictive regulations and policies, the unwillingness of some addicted individuals to enter treatment, the difficulty of linking drug users with the appropriate treatment modality (due to incomplete knowledge of best practices), and insufficient knowledge about treatment services being conducted at the state and local level[6] (ONDCP, 2000c). The discussion below focuses on the first two factors, insufficient funding to provide treatment on request and restrictive policies and regulations regarding methadone treatment, as these are examples of policies driven by underlying social attitudes regarding drug use.

The limited public and private sector financing is a significant factor affecting the availability of drug abuse treatment services (ONDCP, 2000c), particularly for low income and uninsured individuals. Over time, support for drug abuse treatment has led to a distinctly two-tiered treatment system that is distinguished primarily by mode of financing (IOM, 1990). The publicly supported treatment system serves primarily indigent clients, while the private system serves primarily clients with private health insurance or those who can afford to pay for treatment (IOM, 1990; Weisner et al., 1999). Of the estimated $7.6 billion spent on drug abuse treatment in 1996, public-sector spending accounted for approximately $5 billion (66 percent), while private sources accounted for $2.6 billion (34 percent) (McKusick et al., 1998). Of the public-sector funding, non-insurance sources accounted for nearly half (47 percent) of total drug abuse

---

[5]The need for treatment varies according to the severity of the problem. The Department of Health and Human Services has divided those needing treatment into two categories, Level 1 and Level 2, based on intensity of drug use, symptoms, and consequences. Level 2 is the more severe. The 5.1 million individuals reflects Level 2 drug users (ONDCP, 2000c).

[6]A significant amount of federal funding is distributed each year ($1.6 billion in FY 1999) (SAMHSA, 2000) to states through the Substance Abuse Prevention and Treatment (SAPT) block grant to support substance abuse prevention and treatment services. States have broad discretion in how the SAPT block grant funds are distributed (to cities, counties, and service providers), the types of services supported, and the amount allocated to drug treatment services. Presently, little information exists about the effectiveness of drug treatment programs funded by the SAPT block grant. The Substance Abuse and Mental Health Services Administration (SAMHSA), the agency which administers the block grant, primarily monitors states' compliance with the statutory requirements regarding use of funds, but has done little to assess outcomes of these programs. Efforts by SAMHSA and some states are now under way to measure the effectiveness of these programs (GAO, 2000).

treatment spending. These sources included federal block grants (e.g., the SAPT Block Grant), funding from the Department of Veterans Affairs, and the Department of Defense, and funding from state and local governments. Public insurance programs, including Medicaid and Medicare, contributed approximately one-fifth (19 percent) of total drug abuse treatment spending (McKusick et al., 1998).

Recent changes in public and private insurance coverage may have affected access to drug abuse treatment. In 1996, Congress passed legislation that eliminated substance abuse as a primary qualifying diagnosis for federal Supplemental Security Income (SSI) and Social Security Disability Insurance (SSDI) (Goldstein et al., 2000; Swartz et al., 2000). These changes eliminated cash and Medicaid benefits for approximately 250,000 individuals nationwide (Goldstein et al., 2000).[7] According to some observers, this policy change was made largely in response to press reports that federal disability payments were supporting or encouraging drug use (Swartz et al., 2000). Some individuals who were disqualified from SSI or SSDI were able to requalify under another disability category.[8] However, this change eliminated the primary source of coverage for substance abuse treatment services for many low income individuals (Horgan and Hodgkin, 1999). Many former SSI recipients who lost benefits as a result of the change, and who continued to be unemployed or underemployed, had high rates of drug dependence and co-occurring psychiatric disorders (Swartz et al., 2000). These factors were major impediments to finding stable employment. One recent study found that only a small proportion of the sample of former SSI drug and alcohol addicted recipients were able to gain even marginal employment one year after termination of benefits (Swartz et al., 2000).

On the private sector side, the scope of benefits for substance abuse treatment is generally limited and less comprehensive than for other illnesses (Horgan and Hodgkin, 1999). While coverage for inpatient detoxification is generally treated like coverage for other inpatient care, coverage for inpatient rehabilitation and outpatient care is generally more restricted (Bureau of Labor Statistics, 1999, 1998). A recent study found that private insurance coverage for drug abuse treatment has decreased in previous years through the imposition of formal limits, such as restric-

---

[7]Not all of the individuals who lost coverage as a result of this legislation were drug and alcohol dependent. The legislation also established more restrictive SSI/SSDI eligibility standards for children with disabling conditions.

[8]For example, individuals with co-occurring substance abuse and mental health disorders could qualify for Medicaid if they met federal-state income and disability eligibility criteria.

tions on the number of hospital days and outpatient visits, or maximum dollar coverage (McKusick et al., 1998).

Treatment capacity has historically been limited in the public treatment system, particularly in areas with high prevalence of drug abuse. In contrast, the private sector treatment system has reserve capacity in many areas (IOM, 1990). A 1997 Substance Abuse and Mental Health Services Administration (SAMHSA) survey of treatment facilities with residential and inpatient treatment beds suggests similar findings. The survey shows that reserve capacity was lowest in government-owned hospitals and treatment facilities, while reserve capacity was highest among privately-owned treatment facilities (SAMHSA, 1999a).

Federal drug control policy over the past 20 years has contributed to the capacity constraints in the public treatment system. The federal government has provided substantial increases in funding to expand the capacity of prisons for drug offenders, but relatively meager increases for drug abuse treatment (Kleiman, 1992). Indeed, an erosion in federal funding for drug abuse treatment between 1976 and 1987 essentially halted growth in the public treatment sector (IOM, 1990). While the public treatment system remained neglected throughout most of the 1980s, federal investments in the criminal justice system experienced a period of unprecedented growth. Although federal funding for drug abuse treatment has increased over the past decade, the growth rate for drug abuse treatment spending remains much flatter than the growth rate for criminal justice spending (ONDCP, 2000b) (see Figure 7.1).[9] The ongoing capacity constraints in publicly financed treatment settings, however, suggest the need for significant, continued investment.

Government regulations also limit the availability of treatment for those in need. Methadone, in particular, is subject to extensive regulation.[10] At the federal level, methadone is regulated in three ways, making it the nation's most regulated medication. First, the manufacturing, labeling, and dispensing of methadone are subject to Food and Drug Adminis-

---

[9]The significant increase in total drug control spending was primarily due to increased funding for supply-side reduction interventions, which include spending on law enforcement (primarily criminal justice), international supply reduction efforts, and interdiction. Criminal justice system spending accounts for 95 percent of law enforcement spending and 72 percent of total supply reduction spending (ONDCP, 2000b).

[10]While methadone is the most frequently used pharmacotherapy for treating opiate addiction, other chemical modalities, including levo-alpha-acetylmethadol (LAAM), buprenorphine, and naltrexone are also effective. These alternative medications can sometimes offer patients important advantages over methadone. LAAM, for instance, can prevent withdrawal symptoms for up to 96 hours in contrast to the 24 hour period of effectiveness with methadone, reducing the number of required clinic visits (NIH, 1997b).

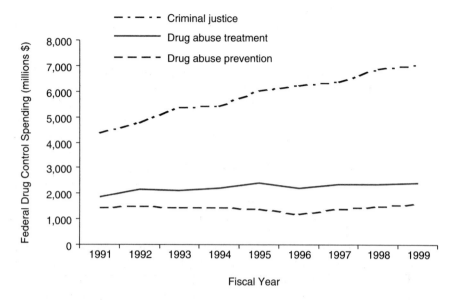

FIGURE 7.1 Federal drug control spending, Fiscal Years 1991–1999. NOTE: Spending reported in 1992 dollars. SOURCE: Nominal drug control expenditure data from the Office of National Drug Control Policy (ONDCP, 2000b). Price deflators were provided by the Bureau of Labor Statistics.

tration (FDA) standards regarding safety, efficacy, and quality of all prescription drugs. Second, it is regulated by the Drug Enforcement Agency under the requirements for schedule II narcotics to prevent diversion and illegal use. Third, methadone is subject to a unique set of regulations, established by the Department of Health and Human Services (DHHS), that controls how and under what circumstances methadone may be used to treat opiate addiction. In addition to federal regulations, methadone is often further restricted by many states, and it is sometimes regulated at the county and municipal level (IOM, 1995b).[11]

These extensive regulations have had several unintended consequences. First, treatment programs are not tailored to individual needs and may provide subtherapeutic doses (Strain et al., 1999; IOM, 1995b; D'Aunno and Vaughn, 1992), thus increasing the likelihood of treatment failure. Second, regulations impose limits on the ability of physicians and

---

[11]The IOM report on Federal Regulation of Methadone (1995b) contains a more detailed discussion of regulations regarding methadone treatment.

other health care professionals to exercise professional judgment in providing methadone maintenance treatment for their patients (IOM, 1995b). Third, isolation of treatment centers from the mainstream medical care system creates barriers to linkages with other ancillary services (e.g., mental health care, medical care) (IOM, 1995b). Fourth, there are economic costs (shared by programs, insurers, patients, and tax payers) associated with assuring compliance with regulatory requirements (IOM, 1995b). Finally, participation in methadone treatment results in a significant loss of patient autonomy and a climate of social control (Kleiman, 1992). Dependence on methadone makes patients vulnerable to threats of or actual withholding of the medication. Many addicts are unwilling to relinquish this autonomy until they are so desperate that they do not have a choice. Many addicts with jobs or other routine daily activities also find the current regulations requiring them to attend methadone clinic on a daily basis too burdensome (IOM, 1995b).

Although this web of regulations was initially developed, in part, in response to reports of abuses of methadone, its primary goal was to address concerns about its illegal diversion (IOM, 1995b). Evidence indicates, however, that the amount of methadone diverted for illicit use is relatively small (IOM, 1995b). The extensive regulation of methadone places too much emphasis on protecting society from methadone itself, rather than from the addiction, violence, and infectious disease morbidity that methadone maintenance treatment can help prevent (IOM, 1995b). Several expert panels (NIH, 1997b; IOM, 1995b) have consequently recommended that current regulations be modified to give greater weight to clinical judgment and to allow for improved access to methadone treatment.[12]

Many of the factors limiting access to or availability of drug abuse treatment are related to several common misperceptions. For example, a recent IOM study noted that one of the most enduring myths related to addiction is that treatment for these disorders is ineffective (IOM, 1997a). However, numerous studies establish addiction as a chronic, relapsing medical condition that can be effectively managed through treatment,[13]

---

[12]On July 22, 1999, the DHHS issued a Notice of Proposed Rulemaking (DHHS, 1999) that would make regulatory changes to improve federal oversight of methadone treatment programs, expand access to treatment, and allow physicians more flexibility in treating opiate addiction outside of the traditional methadone clinic settings. Under the new rule, methadone treatment programs would be accredited under a new program managed by SAMHSA, replacing the 30-year-old inspection program of the FDA (SAMHSA, 1999b). At the time of this report, the proposed rule had not been finalized and the Committee had not evaluated these proposed regulations.

[13]Previous IOM committees have defined drug addiction as a chronic, relapsing brain

with significant benefits accruing to both the individual and society (NIH, 1997b; NRC and IOM, 1995). Other misconceptions appear to flow from the stigma surrounding drug abuse and addiction (NIH, 1997b; IOM, 1997a; IOM, 1998; Drucker et al., 1998). Public attitudes toward addiction are overwhelmingly negative, with many people believing that addiction is simply a moral failing or a self-induced problem resulting from lack of willpower or motivation (NIH, 1997b; IOM, 1997a; IOM, 1995b).

The stigma surrounding drug use also can isolate drug users from medical and social services, such as education, prevention, or drug abuse treatment efforts, that could help reduce the risk of HIV (Drucker et al., 1998). In addition, stigma may limit public support and advocacy for drug abuse treatment. For instance, the "not in my backyard" syndrome has seriously hindered efforts to site drug abuse treatment facilities in new areas (IOM, 1998). Similarly, unlike other chronic diseases, such as cancer or heart disease, which have strong advocacy organizations and patient constituencies arguing for expansion of prevention, treatment, and research, there are few advocates for the drug addicted population (IOM, 1998).

The underlying misperceptions and stigma associated with addiction, drug use, and treatment have shaped policy decisions and public support of efforts to address the twin epidemics of HIV and substance abuse. Previous federal policy largely focused on increasing funding for imprisonment of drug sellers and users, with relatively small increases for drug abuse treatment (Kleiman, 1992). The national policy to incarcerate drug offenders has been a major contributor to the explosive growth in the incarcerated population over the past decade.

There are indications that the federal response may reflect public sentiment. A recent study reviewing 47 national public opinion polls and surveys conducted between 1978 and 1997 showed strong support for criminal justice responses to the drug problem, but relatively weak support for increasing funding for drug abuse treatment. While most Americans (58 percent) do not see the nation's illegal drug problem improving despite significant increases in national spending, they continue to support the same general policy direction as followed in the past (Blendon and Young, 1998).

The Committee believes that drug abuse treatment is an effective, but highly underutilized HIV prevention strategy. However, there is increasing support on the federal level for closing the public drug abuse treatment gap (ONDCP, 2000c; ONDCP, 1999). SAMHSA, the federal agency

---

disease, which is manifested by a complex set of behaviors resulting from genetic, biological, psychosocial, and environmental interactions (IOM, 1997a).

charged with improving the quality and availability of substance abuse and mental health prevention, treatment, and rehabilitation services, has a critical role in leading efforts to address the interrelated epidemics of substance abuse, mental illness, and HIV. In addition, collaborations among a multitude of federal, state, and local agencies and private insurers that fund and administer drug abuse treatment programs will be necessary to reduce the treatment gap and change social and cultural norms and beliefs about drug abuse and addiction.

Therefore, the Committee recommends that:

Federal agencies (including the Substance Abuse and Mental Health Services Administration, the Health Care Financing Administration, the Office of National Drug Control Policy, the Department of Veterans Affairs, and the National Institute on Drug Abuse), state and local agencies, and private insurers that fund, administer, or conduct research on drug abuse treatment programs should collaborate to develop mechanisms to: (1) increase drug treatment resources to the level needed for all of those requesting access; and (2) integrate and link these services with appropriate psychiatric and HIV prevention and treatment services.

Access to Sterile Drug Injection Equipment

Drug abuse treatment is not a panacea for the drug epidemic, however. Regardless of the availability of treatment opportunities, a certain portion of drug users will continue to inject drugs. For those who cannot or will not stop injecting drugs, the one-time use of sterile needles and syringes remains the safest and most effective method for preventing HIV transmission. Indeed, a recent study produced similar results, suggesting that expanded provision of needle exchange programs in the United States could have averted between 10,000 and 20,000 new infections over the past decade (Lurie and Drucker, 1997).

Although many communities and law enforcement officials have expressed concern that increasing availability of injection equipment will lead to increased drug use, criminal activity, and discarded contaminated syringes, studies have found no scientifically reliable evidence of these negative effects (GAO, 1993). Studies also have shown that needle exchange programs serve as an important link to other medical and social services, particularly drug abuse treatment and counseling programs (Lurie and Reingold, 1993; Heimer, 1998). A review by the National Research Council and the Institute of Medicine concluded that needle exchange programs reduced risk behaviors, such as multi-person reuse of syringes, by 80 percent and led to reductions in HIV transmission of 30 percent or more (NRC and IOM, 1995). A study of a needle exchange program in New Haven, Connecticut, estimated that the program led to a 33 percent reduction in HIV infection rates among drug users, without any increase in the level of substance abuse (Kaplan and O'Keefe, 1993; Kaplan, 1995). Similarly, in 1992, the partial repeal of syringe prescription and drug paraphernalia laws in Connecticut increased IDUs' access to sterile syringes (Valleroy et al., 1995). Fewer IDUs reported purchasing syringes on the street after the change (74 percent before versus 28 percent after). Among IDUs who reported ever sharing a syringe, syringe sharing also declined after the new laws (52 percent before versus 31 percent after) (Groseclose et al., 1995).

Despite such compelling empirical evidence, however, states and the federal government limit the availability of sterile injection equipment through a series of legal and funding mechanisms (Gostin, 1998). All 50 states have laws that restrict the sale, distribution, and/or possession of injection equipment: 49 states have drug paraphernalia laws that prohibit the manufacture, sale, distribution, possession, or advertisement of any device, including syringes, that may be used in preparing or injecting illicit drugs; and 14 states have syringe prescription laws that require a medical prescription for the sale or possession of injection equipment (Burris et al., 2000). As of 1997, 23 states had pharmacy regulations that limited the ability of pharmacists to dispense injection equipment without verification that its use has a valid medical purpose (Gostin et al., 1997). In addition, the federal Mail Order Drug Paraphernalia Act prohibits sale and transportation of syringes and other drug paraphernalia in interstate commerce (Gostin, 1998).

In addition, a series of statutes enacted by Congress since 1988 specifically prohibit the use of federal funds to support needle exchange programs, regardless of whether or not programs are legally authorized by the individual state. Under the fiscal year 1998 U.S. Department of Health and Human Services Appropriation Act (P.L. 105-78), however, the federal funding ban could be lifted if the Secretary of Health and Human Services determined that needle exchange programs were effective in preventing the spread of HIV and did not encourage illicit drug use. Based on findings from a number of expert review panels and federally funded studies, Secretary Donna E. Shalala announced on April 20, 1998, that there was sufficient empirical evidence to meet this two-pronged test (DHHS, 1998). Despite the Secretary's finding, however, the Administration did not rescind the ban—largely out of political concerns, according to some observers—(Stolberg, 1998) opting instead to allow local communities to implement their own needle exchange programs, using their own resources to fund them (DHHS, 1998).

These legal and funding restrictions limit syringe access in several ways. First, prescription laws and pharmacy regulations limit the ability of pharmacists to dispense syringes over the counter. In addition, drug paraphernalia laws limit the willingness of injection drug users to adopt safer injection practices (e.g., carrying their own injection equipment) out of fear of arrest or prosecution. Finally, syringe prescription laws limit the legal establishment and operation of needle exchange programs, and funding restrictions limit the financial capability of these programs to operate. Although the number of reported needle exchange programs has increased over the past several years (CDC, 1998), these restrictions still severely restrict the number of these programs. As of May 2000, an estimated 156 needle exchange programs were in operation in the United States (NASEN, personal communication).

The Committee believes that improving access to sterile injection equipment is a critical component of HIV prevention. Therefore, the Committee recommends that:

> **Legal barriers to the purchase and possession of injection equipment should be removed, including repeal of state prescription laws and modification of state and local drug paraphernalia laws. In addition, the Administration should rescind the existing prohibition against the use of federal funds for needle exchange to allow communities that desire such programs to institute them using federal resources.**

Comprehensive Sex Education and Condom Availability in Schools

Teenagers and young adults are at increasing risk for acquiring HIV. In 1998, AIDS was the ninth leading cause of death among youth ages 15–24, and the fifth leading cause of death among individuals 25–44, many of whom were infected as teenagers (Murphy, 2000). The majority of infections among adolescents and young adults are sexually transmitted (CDC, 2000a). Adolescents are at higher risk for acquiring HIV than adults for several reasons: they are more likely to have multiple (either sequential or concurrent) sexual partners, they are more likely to engage in unprotected sex, and they are more likely to select partners at higher risk (CDC, 1999c). These high-risk behaviors also place youth at increased risk for other STDs and for unintended pregnancy. Indeed, the United States has the highest teenage pregnancy rate of all developed countries (CDC, 2000b), and over 3 million teenagers acquire an STD in any given year (IOM, 1997b). In light of these facts, youth constitute an extremely important population for HIV, STD, and pregnancy prevention efforts.

The school setting is an obvious venue for providing such information, given that nearly 95 percent of all youth ages 5–17 years are enrolled in primary and secondary schools (Department of Education, 2000). To a large extent, policies regarding sex education and condom availability in schools are determined by state mandates and by policies established within local school districts. As a result, the specific content of sex education and condom availability programs varies substantially across school districts. In general, sex education curricula fall into two broad categories: those that teach an abstinence-only message, and those with a comprehensive message. Abstinence-only programs teach abstinence outside of marriage as the only option, with discussions of contraception either entirely prohibited or limited to its shortcomings. In contrast, comprehensive sex education programs provide information about abstinence in the context of a broader sexuality education program, and they also may make condoms available to students. Also included under the rubric of programs with a comprehensive sexual health and education message are "abstinence-plus" programs that teach abstinence as the preferred option for adolescents, but also permit discussion of contraception, pregnancy, and disease prevention (Kaiser Family Foundation, 1999b).

Decisions regarding the content of sex education curricula and whether or not to make condoms available at schools have been the focus of considerable debate and controversy. Proponents of abstinence-only policies argue that providing information about contraception or providing condoms to adolescents sends a mixed message to youth and may promote sexual activity (e.g., accelerating the onset of sexual intercourse and increasing the frequency of sexual intercourse or number of sexual partners) (Kaiser Family Foundation, 1999b). Proponents of comprehensive programs argue that while abstinence should be encouraged until youth are emotionally and physically ready for sex, it is crucial to provide youth who may be sexually active with information and contraceptive methods that can protect them from STDs and unintended pregnancy (Kaiser Family Foundation, 1999b).

Studies reviewing the scientific literature, as well as expert panels that have studied this issue, have concluded that comprehensive sex and HIV/AIDS education programs[14] and condom availability programs can be effective in reducing high-risk sexual behaviors among adolescents

---

[14]In a comprehensive review of school-based sex education programs, Kirby (2000) concludes that nearly all evaluations of sex and AIDS education programs demonstrate some socially desirable outcome, such as an increase in knowledge. Furthermore, some studies have provided scientifically credible evidence of reductions in risky sexual behavior. However, other studies did not demonstrate such impacts on behavior. The author identified 10 characteristics of programs that may distinguish effective programs from ineffective ones.

(Kirby, 2000; IOM, 1997b; IOM, 1995a; Kirby, 1995). In addition, these reviews and expert panels conclude that school-based sex education and condom availability programs do not increase sexual activity among adolescents.

National surveys show strong public support for comprehensive sex education policies and condom availability programs. A 1998 poll found that 81 percent of adults supported schools teaching information about abstinence as well as about contraception and prevention of STDs (Kaiser Family Foundation, 1998). A 1991 poll showed that 64 percent of adults favored making condoms available in high schools (Roper Organization, 1991), and a 1999 poll found that 53 percent of adults thought school personnel should make condoms available to sexually active youth (Haffner and Wagoner, 1999). Condom availability programs are also endorsed by the American Academy of Pediatrics (AAP, 1995).

In contrast, two recent reviews of the literature on abstinence-only education programs concluded that the evidence was insufficient to determine whether abstinence programs decrease sexual activity (Kirby, 2000; Maynard, 2000). One of these reviews concluded that the weight of the evidence indicated that abstinence programs do not delay the onset of intercourse, but significant methodological limitations could have obscured the impact of these interventions (Kirby, 2000). Public support for abstinence-only education programs is also limited. In a 1998 poll, only 18 percent of adults thought abstinence should be the only topic of discussion (Kaiser Family Foundation, 1998).

Still, many school districts do not provide comprehensive programs. A 1998 national survey found that of school districts with a policy to teach sex education, only two-thirds permitted positive discussions of contraception (Landry et al., 1999). In addition, a 1995 survey found that only 2.2 percent of all public high schools and 0.3 percent of school districts made condoms available to students (Kirby and Brown, 1996).

In contrast, abstinence-only programs have proliferated. A 1998 survey found that one-third of all school districts with a policy to teach sex education used abstinence-only education that prohibited dissemination of any positive information about contraception (Landry et al., 1999). This study found that every region of the country had a significant proportion of districts with abstinence-only policies; however, districts in the South were five times as likely as those in the Northeast to have an abstinence-only policy. The survey also found that among those districts that changed their sex education policies, twice as many adopted a more abstinence-focused policy than vice versa (Landry et al., 1999).

While federal involvement in sex education has historically been limited, two federal programs provide sizeable amounts of funding for abstinence-only sex education programs: the 1981 Adolescent Family Life Act

(AFLA) and the 1996 Personal Responsibility and Work Opportunity Reconciliation Act (PRWORA) (42 U.S.C.A. §§ 601 et seq.). The AFLA, which provides funds for abstinence-only sex education under Title XX of the Public Health Service Act, was enacted by Congress with the primary goal of preventing teenage pregnancy by promoting abstinence education, providing care for pregnant and parenting teens, and conducting research on teen sexuality. Since 1982, an estimated $60 million has been spent on some form of abstinence education through AFLA, although no exact figures are available (Kaiser Family Foundation, 1999c). The PRWORA, which was part of the 1996 welfare reform law, provides states with a total of $50 million annually for five years, from FY1998 through FY2002, to support abstinence-unless-married education programs.[15] States that accept federal funding are required to provide 75 percent in matching funds, resulting in a total of as much as $87.5 million per year ($437.5 million over five years) for abstinence-only programs. By FY99, all 50 states, Puerto Rico, and the Virgin Islands had applied for and received funding under PRWORA for abstinence-only education. Recent reviews show that states use their funds for a wide array of programs, including school- and community-based programs (SIECUS, 1999). A national evaluation of this initiative is currently being conducted using funds allocated as a part of the Balanced Budget Act of 1997, and many states are undertaking separate evaluations of their programs (AMCHP, 1999).

The Committee believes that investing hundreds of millions of dollars of federal and state funds over five years in abstinence-only programs with no evidence of effectiveness constitutes poor fiscal and public health policy. The Committee concurs with the prior conclusion of the National Institutes of Health Consensus Panel on Interventions to Prevent HIV Risk Behaviors (NIH, 1997b): that legislative restrictions discouraging ef-

---

[15]The law defines an abstinence education program as having eight components that teach:

- abstinence has social, psychological, and health benefits;
- unmarried, school-aged children are expected to abstain from sex;
- abstinence is the only certain way to prevent out-of-wedlock pregnancy and STDs;
- a mutually faithful monogamous married relationship is the standard for sexual activity;
- sexual activity outside marriage is likely to have harmful psychological and physical effects;
- out-of-wedlock childbearing is likely to harm the child, the parents, and society;
- how to reject sexual advances and how alcohol and drug use increases vulnerability to them; and
- the importance of attaining self-sufficiency before engaging in sex.

SOURCE: Kaiser Family Foundation, 1999b.

fective programs aimed at youth must be eliminated, and that programs must include information about safer sex behaviors, including condom use.

Therefore, the Committee recommends that:

Congress, as well as other federal, state, and local policymakers, eliminate requirements that public funds be used for abstinence-only education, and that states and local school districts implement and continue to support age-appropriate comprehensive sex education and condom availability programs in schools.

HIV Prevention in Correctional Settings

Approximately 6.3 million adults were under the supervision of federal, state, and local correctional authorities in 1999 in the United States. An estimated 1.9 million of these individuals were incarcerated in prisons and jails (Beck, 2000), and approximately 4.4 million of them were on probation or parole (Bureau of Justice Statistics, 2000). Most inmates come from low-income urban areas, and minorities are disproportionately represented among inmates. Many inmates have a history of substance use or sexual behaviors that place them at high risk for HIV infection, (Hammett et al., 1998; Braithewaite et al., 1996), as well as for STDs, tuberculosis, hepatitis, and other health problems (Hammett et al., 1998; Dean-Gaitor and Fleming, 1999). A recent survey estimated that in 1997, AIDS prevalence was five times higher, and HIV prevalence was eight to ten times higher, in prisons and jails than in the general population[16] (Hammett et al., 1999). As a result, the correctional system constitutes a critical setting for HIV prevention and treatment interventions. The benefits of such efforts will extend beyond the correctional system as well, since the circulation of infected or high risk individuals between correctional facilities and communities is a dynamic that now helps maintain the epidemic and contributes to new cases each year in many urban areas (Braithewaite et al., 1996).

The primary barrier to implementing HIV prevention programs and strategies in correctional settings is the difference in priorities between public health officials and correctional system officials. The public health community's primary focus is to improve the health of inmates and to protect the community to which they return from the spread of infection.

---

[16]In the absence of a mandatory HIV testing policy, no precise data exist on the prevalence or incidence of HIV or AIDS in correctional settings. These figures reflect estimates only.

Thus, public health officials tend to advocate strategies that, by default, acknowledge the occurrence of sexual activities and drug use in correctional settings. Conversely, the primary focus of correctional officers is to ensure a controlled and secure environment. To do so, they must uphold the policies and regulations of the correctional system that expressly forbids those same activities.

Implementing acceptable HIV prevention strategies in the correctional system will require extensive collaborations among correctional systems, public health officials, and community-based organizations, and developing these collaborations will require significant effort and cooperation by all parties involved. However, failure to address HIV prevention needs in prisons and jails is a shortsighted strategy that will lead to unnecessary new infections and wasted expenditures. There are four primary routes for addressing this issue: helping inmates when they are released, providing HIV/AIDS education to inmates, providing drug abuse treatment in correctional settings, and implementing harm reduction programs.

Discharge Planning

Many inmates, particularly those with a history of substance abuse, have difficulty successfully transitioning from correctional settings to the community. The transition can be especially difficult for inmates with HIV/AIDS, given their increased needs for health care and support services. Discharge planning is critical for these populations, as it facilitates linkages with appropriate public health and community-based resources for follow-up care, treatment, and support services (Hammett et al., 1998).

Although most correctional systems report some type of discharge planning for HIV-infected inmates, only three-fourths of federal and state systems actually make referrals and less than one-third arrange follow-up appointments for inmates for HIV medications, HIV counseling, Medicaid and related benefits, and other types of services or support (Hammett et al., 1999) (see Table 7.1). Several other barriers hinder the smooth transition of inmates into the community. Many inmates are incarcerated in correctional facilities far from their homes, thus making it more difficult to facilitate linkages to community services in their cities of residence (National Center on Addiction and Substance Abuse, 1998). Existing community programs may lack the capacity to provide the necessary prevention, care, and support services to new clients; additionally, waiting lists, limited placements, and increasing demands for certain types of services (e.g., substance abuse treatment) bring unwanted delays to those in need. Other factors—such as staffing constraints, lack of cooperation between the criminal justice system and community organizations, difficulty in maintaining accurate records, and communication difficulties—are also

TABLE 7.1 HIV/AIDS Education, Harm Reduction, and Discharge Planning Programs in U.S. Adult Correctional Systems, 1997

	State/Federal Prison Systems (N = 51)		City/County Jail Systems (N = 41)	
	N	%	N	%
Type of HIV Education Programs				
Instructor-Led Education		94		73
"Comprehensive" HIV/AIDS education programs*		10		5
Topics Covered in HIV Education Programs				
Basic HIV information	51	100	35	85
Meaning of HIV test results	51	100	38	93
Negotiation skills for safer sex	21	41	19	46
Safer injection practices	23	45	20	49
Tattooing risks	42	82	22	54
Alcohol/drug risks	41	80	30	73
Self-perception of risk	30	59	27	66
Identifying barriers to behavioral change	28	55	23	56
Harm Reduction Strategies				
Make condoms available	2	4	4	10
Make bleach available (for any purpose)	10	20	8	20
Make needles/syringe equipment available	0	0	0	0

	Percentage of State/Federal Prison Systems Providing (N = 51)		Percentage of City/County Jail Systems Providing (N = 41)	
Discharge planning services for HIV+ inmates	92		76	
	Referral Made	Appointment Made	Referral Made	Appointment Made
Medicaid/related benefits	78	35	56	29
CD4 monitoring	71	24	54	17
Viral load monitoring	61	22	46	20
HIV medications	82	31	66	27
Substance abuse treatment	75	22	63	24
HIV counseling	73	27	61	32
Psychosocial support	73	24	54	27
STD prevention and treatment	65	22	46	17

*Provides all of the following in all of its facilities: instructor-led education, peer-led programs, pre-/posttest counseling, and multisession prevention counseling.

SOURCE: NIJ et al., 1999.

impediments to effective transitions between correctional systems and the community (HRSA, 1995).

Several correctional facilities, however, have developed promising models for improving discharge planning and continuity of care for inmates upon their return to the community. Seven programs, jointly funded by the CDC and Ryan White CARE Act's Special Projects of National Significance in fiscal year 1999 and fiscal year 2000, provided comprehensive HIV education and transitional services for inmates. Evaluations of these programs have identified six key elements of success: case management, staff skills and training, intra- and interagency referral, client participation in discharge planning, use of former inmates as service providers, and recognition of HIV as a problem by correctional facilities and community agencies (HRSA, 1995).

One model program, funded by the CDC and HRSA, for example, was developed by the Hampden County Correctional Center in Massachusetts. This comprehensive HIV program includes case management and discharge planning components to link infected inmates with health care services upon their release. Releasees are also linked into agencies that can assist them with other concerns, such as housing and employment. This program has shown initial signs of success: in 1997, more than 70 percent of persons with HIV/AIDS who had been released kept their appointments (NIJ et al., 1999).

HIV Prevention Education

While all state and federal prison systems offer basic HIV information and instruction on the meaning of an HIV test result, only two-thirds of the systems provide information on safer sex practices, and less than half teach safer sex negotiation skills or provide information about safer drug injection practices (see Table 7.1). Only 10 percent of prisons and 5 percent of jails currently offer comprehensive programs of instructor- and peer-led education, pre- and posttest counseling, and multisession prevention counseling (Hammett et al., 1999).

This failure to provide adequate education stems from the hesitancy of correctional facility administrators to acknowledge or accept that high-risk behaviors occur within the correctional system. Because sexual activity and injection drug use are illegal in prisons and jails, many seem to believe that teaching preventive behaviors will be viewed as condoning illegal practices (Braithewaite et al., 1996). Even if inmates are not engaging in risk behaviors while incarcerated, instruction in safer sexual and drug use behavior would be beneficial for when they are released into their communities.

Drug Abuse Treatment

There is a high prevalence of substance abuse problems among incarcerated populations. A 1997 survey found that more than 80 percent of state prisoners and more than 70 percent of federal prisoners reported past drug use, more than 40 percent of federal prisoners reported using drugs in the month prior to their offense, and one-quarter of state prisoners and one-sixth of federal prisoners indicated past alcohol or substance abuse or dependence. Further, one in six state and federal prisoners reported the need for drug money as the reason for the crime that led to his or her incarceration, and one-third of state prisoners and one-fifth of federal prisoners reported using drugs at the time of their offense (Mumola, 1999). Many substance-using criminal offenders under the control of the criminal justice system are not incarcerated, but are on parole, probation, or other supervised arrangements in the general community. Many of these individuals are poorly supervised, lack employment or health insurance coverage, and often relapse into substance use or other risk behaviors (Pollack et al., 1999).[17]

However it has been estimated that only 18 to 25 percent of inmates in need of treatment are actually receiving it (Mumola, 1999; National Center on Addiction and Substance Abuse, 1998). A recent study of women's prisons also found long waiting lists for residential drug abuse treatment programs (GAO, 1999). In a 1997 survey, federal correctional facilities were the most likely to provide drug treatment (94 percent), followed by approximately 56 percent of state facilities, and 33 percent of local facilities. Approximately 173,000 inmates received substance abuse treatment, with 70 percent receiving treatment or counseling in the general facility population, 28 percent receiving treatment in specialized substance abuse treatment facilities within the institution, and 2 percent receiving treatment in an inpatient hospital/psychiatric setting (SAMHSA, 1999b).[18]

In a 1996 survey conducted by the Federal Bureau of Justice and correctional systems in 47 states and Washington, D.C., 75 percent of systems cited budgetary constraints as the main reason why they did not offer drug treatment (National Center on Addiction and Substance Abuse, 1998). Another study identified additional barriers, including a limited number of substance abuse counselors, frequent movement of inmates, general correctional problems, problems with aftercare provision, and

---

[17]See Pollack et al. (1999) for a discussion of health care delivery and substance abuse treatment strategies for probationers, parolees, and other offenders in the general community.

[18]Data on the number of inmates receiving methadone maintenance treatment were not reported.

legislative mandates (National Center on Addiction and Substance Abuse, 1998). This study also found that prisoners with substance abuse problems may be reluctant to participate in drug treatment programs. Their reluctance was attributed to other aspects of correctional life (e.g., increased sentences if they admit drug abuse problems, few incentives for early release or parole, and lack of rehabilitative programs) that contributed to feelings of despair and loss of personal empowerment. Thus, it is important to address the multiple needs that substance abusers may have if treatment is to be accepted and effective.

Not all correctional facilities can realistically offer drug treatment services to inmates. For instance, juvenile detention centers and local jails may hold offenders for only a few days. State and federal prisons, which house inmates with longer sentences, have a greater responsibility and capacity to offer substance abuse treatment to their inmates.

Harm Reduction Programs

Harm reduction strategies, including making condoms, needles or syringes, or bleach which can be used to clean needles and syringes,[19] available to inmates, have not been widely adopted in U.S. correctional facilities (see Table 7.1). This lack is due to two major factors. First, needles and bleach constitute a serious safety concern in correctional settings, and condoms can be used for smuggling drugs or contraband. The second factor is the apparent belief among most correctional officials that implementing measures targeted at these behaviors would essentially condone them (Hammett et al., 1998). The existence of antisodomy statutes may pose an additional barrier to the implementation of condom availability programs in some states.

According to a 1997 national survey conducted for the National Institute of Justice and the CDC, two state correctional systems (Vermont and Mississippi) and four municipal jail systems (New York City, Philadelphia, Washington, D.C., and San Francisco) have provided condoms to their inmates. In addition, the six state or federal prison systems that permitted conjugal visits (as of 1997) also made condoms available to inmates participating in these visits (NIJ et al., 1999). In contrast, condoms are available in most European and Canadian prisons, and condom distribution pilot programs have been initiated in Australia (NIJ et al., 1999).

Correctional facilities with condom distribution programs have re-

---

[19]Research suggests that bleach may not be effective for HIV disinfection and is a much less desirable risk reduction strategy than using sterile injection equipment (NRC and IOM, 1995).

ported relatively few problems with use of condoms as weapons or for smuggling contraband (NIJ et al., 1999). In the 1997 survey of facilities, an official at the Mississippi State Prison in Parchman cited only one incident when a condom was used for smuggling (NIJ et al., 1999). In Vermont, officials report that after an initial period of controversy, condom distribution became routine and was no longer an issue. Vermont officials report few problems with the misuse of condoms, and they have observed no evidence that condom distribution has led to an increase in sexual activity or undesirable behavior (NIJ et al., 1999; Braithewaite et al., 1996). In a survey of over 400 correctional officers in Canada's federal prison system, 82 percent reported that condom availability had created no problems in their facilities (NIJ et al., 1999).

While some U.S. correctional facilities provide information about safer drug injection practices, no facilities distribute needles or injection equipment (Hammett et al., 1999; NIJ et al., 1999). Indeed, possession of needles and syringes is illegal in correctional settings (NIJ et al., 1999). Needle exchange programs have, however, been implemented in prison systems in other countries, with considerable success. Switzerland was the first country to introduce prison needle exchange programs, beginning in 1992. Evaluation of such a needle exchange program in the Hindelbank women's facility found that the program did not increase drug consumption and significantly reduced the frequency of needle sharing. In addition, there were no reports of needles being used as weapons, and there were no new cases of HIV or hepatitis B reported among program participants. Based on the experience in Swiss facilities, needle exchange programs have been initiated in several prisons in Germany and in at least one prison in Spain. Plans to initiate a pilot needle exchange program in Australia have also been made (NIJ et al., 1999).

Availability of bleach for cleaning injection equipment is also limited in U.S. prisons. Only one facility (San Francisco) has reported making bleach available expressly for cleaning injection equipment (NIJ and CDC, 1995). However, ten state or federal and eight city or county correctional systems report making bleach available to inmates for general purposes (Hammett et al., 1999; NIJ et al., 1999). Bleach is made more widely available in prisons in other countries. Over half of 20 European systems that responded to the 1997 NIJ/CDC survey reported having such policies. A successful pilot study of a bleach kit distribution program in Canada led to the expansion of this program in all Canadian federal facilities (NIJ et al., 1999).

Therefore, the Committee recommends that:

The Department of Health and Human Services should collaborate with the Department of Justice to develop guidelines

to remove policy barriers that hinder the implementation of effective HIV prevention efforts in correctional settings. At a minimum, these guidelines should ensure that:

- discharge planning is enhanced so that individuals with HIV or who are at high risk for HIV (e.g., due to substance abuse or mental health issues) are linked with appropriate community-based prevention and treatment services;
- comprehensive HIV prevention education programs for incarcerated individuals and staff are implemented in all correctional settings; and
- drug treatment is available for inmates with drug abuse problems.

While there is not yet definitive evidence that condom distribution in correctional facilities would reduce HIV transmission, in light of the absence of problems reported by facilities that have implemented such programs, the Committee recommends that condoms be made readily available to incarcerated individuals.

The Committee recognizes that data on HIV sexual transmission in correctional facilities are lacking, as is evidence that condom availability reduces the incidence of sexually transmitted HIV in these settings. Nonetheless, the Committee concludes that providing condoms to inmates is prudent public health practice for the following reasons. First, condoms are clearly the best available means to reduce the risk of sexually transmitting or acquiring HIV among at-risk individuals having intercourse (Davis and Weller, 1999; Pinkerton and Abramson, 1997). Second, studies have documented higher rates of HIV/AIDS among inmates than in the general population (Hammett et al., 1999). Third, the risk of sexual transmission of HIV in correctional facilities is possible because there is evidence (cited in Braithwaite et al., 1996) indicating that sexual activity does occur in correctional settings despite prohibitions against these activities. Finally, correctional facilities in the United States and other countries that have implemented condom distribution programs have reported relatively few logistical or security problems as a result of such programs (NIJ et al., 1999). The Committee further reasons that providing condoms is a very inexpensive intervention. Based on this evidence, the Committee concludes that in the absence of this intervention, inmates are at increased risk of transmitting or acquiring HIV.

The Committee is not making a recommendation at this time with regard to needle availability in correctional settings. The Committee recognizes that lack of access to sterile injection equipment and/or bleach in correctional facilities may result in fewer averted infections, but we understand the concerns of the correctional system with regard to safety threats (both to corrections staff and other inmates) that could result from making these items available to inmates. However, in the absence of these measures, the Committee believes that HIV educational programs in correctional facilities should include information about safe injection practices and all inmates needing substance abuse treatment should receive such services upon request.

REFERENCES

Abdool Karim Q, Tarantola D, As Sy E, Moodie R. 1998. Government responses to HIV/AIDS in Africa: what have we learnt? *AIDS* 11(Suppl B):S143–S149.

American Academy of Pediatrics (AAP). 1995. Condom availability for youth [Web Page]. Located at: www.aap.org/policy/00654.html.

Association of Maternal and Child Health Programs (AMCHP). 1999. *Abstinence Education in the States—Implementation of the 1996 Abstinence Education Law*. Washington, DC: AMCHP.

Association of Reproductive Health, Association of Nurse Practitioners in Reproductive Health (ARHP and ANPRH). 1995. STD counseling and practices and needs survey. Silver Spring, MD: Schulman, Roca, and Bucuvalas, Inc.

Ball JC, Lange WR, Myers CP, Friedman SR. 1988. Reducing the risk of AIDS through methadone maintenance treatment. *Journal of Health and Social Behavior* 29(3):214–226.

Bayne–Smith M. (Ed.). 1996. *Race, Gender, and Health. Sage Series on Race and Ethnic Relations*, Vol. 15. Thousand Oaks, CA: Sage Publications.

Beck A. 2000. Prison and jail inmates at midyear 1999. Bureau of Justice Statistics Bulletin. Washington, DC: U.S. Department of Justice, Office of Justice Programs.

Blendon RJ and Young JT. 1998. The public and the war on illicit drugs. *Journal of the American Medical Association* 279(11):827–832.

Braithewaite RL, Hammett TM, Mayberry RM. 1996. *Prisons and AIDS: A Public Health Challenge*. San Francisco: Jossey–Bass.

Broome KM, Joe GW, Simpson DD. 1999. HIV risk reduction in outpatient drug abuse treatment: Individual and geographic differences. *AIDS Education and Prevention* 11(4):293–306.

Bureau of Justice Statistics. 2000. U.S. correctional population reaches 6.3 million men and women represents 3.1 percent of the adults U.S. population (Press release). Washington, DC.

Bureau of Labor Statistics. 1999. Employee Benefits in Medium and Large Private Establishments, 1997, Bulletin 2517. Washington, DC.

Bureau of Labor Statistics. 1998. Employee Benefits in Medium and Large Private Establishments, 1995, Bulletin 2496. Washington, DC.

Burris S, Lurie P, Abrahamson D, Rich JD. 2000. Physician prescribing of sterile injection equipment to prevent HIV infection: time for action. *Annals of Internal Medicine* 133(3):218–226.

Camacho LM, Bartholomew NG, Joe GW, Cloud MA, Simpson DD. 1996. Gender, cocaine and during-treatment HIV risk reduction among injection opioid users in methadone maintenance. *Drug and Alcohol Dependency* 41(1):1–7.

Campbell CA. 1995. Male gender roles and sexuality: Implications for women's AIDS risk and prevention. *Social Science and Medicine* 41(2):197–210.

Centers for Disease Control and Prevention (CDC). 2000a. *HIV/AIDS Surveillance Report, 1999.* 11(2). Atlanta: CDC.

Centers for Disease Control and Prevention (CDC). 2000b. National Center for Chronic Disease and Health Promotion. Teen Pregnancy [Web Page]. Located at: www.CDC.gov/nccdphp/teen.htm.

Centers for Disease Control and Prevention (CDC). 1999a. Increases in unsafe sex and rectal gonorrhea among men who have sex with men—San Francisco, California, 1994–1997. *Morbidity and Mortality Weekly Report* 48(3):45–48.

Centers for Disease Control and Prevention (CDC). 1999b. Resurgent bacterial sexually transmitted disease among men who have sex with men—King county, Washington, 1997–1999. *Morbidity Mortality and Weekly Report* 48(35):773–777.

Centers for Disease Control and Prevention (CDC). 1999c. *Sexually Transmitted Disease Surveillance.* Atlanta: CDC.

Centers for Disease Control and Prevention (CDC). 1998. Update: Syringe exchange programs—United States, 1997. *Morbidity and Mortality Weekly Report* 47(31):652–655.

Centers for Disease Control and Prevention Advisory Committee for HIV and STD Prevention (CDC Advisory Committee). 1999. Work Group Report on HIV Prevention Activities at CDC.

Chesney M and Smith A. 1999. Critical delays in HIV testing and care: The potential role of stigma. *American Behavioral Scientist* 42(7):1162–1174.

Cohen HW and Northridge ME. 2000. Getting political: Racism and urban health. *American Journal of Public Health* 90(6):841–842.

Cohen M, Deamant C, Barkan S, Richardson J, Young M, Holman S, Anastos K, Cohen J, Melnick S. 2000. Domestic violence and childhood sexual abuse in HIV-infected women and women at risk for HIV. *American Journal of Public Health* 90(4):560–565.

D'Aunno T and Vaughn TE. 1992. Variations in methadone treatment practices. Results from a national study. *Journal of the American Medical Association* 267(2):253–258.

D'Aunno T, Vaughn TE, McElroy P. 1999. An institutional analysis of HIV prevention efforts by the nation's outpatient drug abuse treatment units. *Journal of Health and Social Behavior* 40(2):175–192.

Davis KR and Weller SC. 1999. The effectiveness of condoms in reducing heterosexual transmission of HIV. *Family Planning Perspectives* 31(6):272–279.

Dean-Gaitor HD and Fleming PL. 1999. Epidemiology of AIDS in incarcerated persons in the United States, 1994–1996. *AIDS* 13(17):2429–2435.

Department of Education, National Center for Education Statistics. 2000. *Digest of Education Statistics, 1999.* Washington, DC: Department of Education.

Department of Health and Human Services, Coordinating Group on HIV/AIDS. 1994. HIV Prevention Work Group Recommendations. Report to Philip Lee and Patsy Fleming. Washington, DC: DHHS.

Department of Health and Human Services. 1998. Research Shows Needle Exchange Programs Reduce HIV Infections without Increasing Drug Use. Press Release, April 20.

Department of Health and Human Services, Food and Drug Administration. 1999. Narcotic drugs in maintenance and detoxification treatment of narcotic dependence: repeal of current regulations and proposal to adopt new regulations; proposed rule. *Federal Register* 64(110):39810–39844.

Dolcini MM, Catania JA, Choi KH, Fullilove MT, Coates TJ. 1996. Cognitive and emotional assessments of perceived risk for HIV among unmarried heterosexuals. *AIDS Education and Prevention* 8(4):294–307.

Drucker E, Lurie P, Wodak A, Alcabes P. 1998. Measuring harm reduction: The effects of needle and syringe exchange programs and methadone maintenance on the ecology of HIV. *AIDS* 12 (Suppl A):S217–S230.

Fife D and Mode C. 1992. AIDS incidence and income. *Journal of Acquired Immune Deficiency Syndromes* 5(11):1105–1110.

Fisher J and Fisher W. 1992. Changing AIDS–risk behavior. *Psychological Bulletin.* 111(3):455–474.

Ford K and Norris AE. 1993. Knowledge of AIDS transmission, risk behavior, and perceptions of risk among urban, low-income, African-American and Hispanic youth. *American Journal of Preventive Medicine* 9(5):297–306.

Fordyce E, Shum R, Pal Singh T, Forlenza S. 1998. Economic and geographic diversity in AIDS incidence among HIV exposure groups in New York City: 1983 to 1995. *AIDS and Public Policy Journal* 13(3):103–114.

Friedman PD, D'Aunno TA, Jin L, Alexander JA. 2000. Medical and psychosocial services in drug abuse treatment: Do stronger linkages promote client utilization? *Health Services Research* 35(2):443–465.

General Accounting Office. 2000. *Drug Abuse Treatment: Efforts Under Way to Determine Effectiveness of State Programs.* Washington, DC: GAO.

General Accounting Office. 1999. *Women in Prison: Issues and Challenges Confronting U.S. Correctional Systems* (GAO/GGS-00-22). Washington, DC: GAO.

General Accounting Office. 1998. *Drug Abuse: Research Shows Treatment Is Effective but Benefits May Be Overstated* (GAO/HEHS-98-72). Washington, DC: GAO.

General Accounting Office. 1993. *Needle Exchange Programs: Research Suggests Promise as an AIDS Prevention Strategy* (GAO/HRD-93-60). Washington, DC: GAO.

Geronimus AT. 2000. To mitigate, resist, or undo: Addressing structural influences on the health of urban populations. *American Journal of Public Health* 90(6):867–872.

Gerrard M. 1982. Sex, sex guilt, and contraceptive use. *Journal of Personality and Social Psychology* 42(1):153–158.

Gerrard M. 1987. Sex, sex guilt and contraceptive use revisited: The 1980's. *Journal of Personality and Social Psychology* 52:975.

Goldstein PJ, Anderson T, Swartz J. 2000. Modes of adaptation to termination of the SSI/SSDI addiction disability: Hustlers, good citizens, and lost souls. *Advances in Medical Sociology* 7:215–238.

Gostin LO, Lazzarini Z, Jones TS, Flaherty K. 1997. Prevention of HIV/AIDS and other blood-borne diseases among injection drug users. A national survey on the regulation of syringes and needles. *Journal of the American Medical Association* 277(1):53–62.

Gostin L. 1998. The legal environment impeding access to sterile syringes and needles: The conflict between law enforcement and public health. *Journal of Acquired Immune Deficiency Syndromes and Human Retrovirology* 18(Suppl 1):S60–S70.

Groseclose SL, Weinstein B, Jones TS, Valleroy LA, Fehrs LJ, Kassler WJ. 1995. Impact of increased legal access to needles and syringes on practices of injecting-drug users and police officers—Connecticut, 1992–1993. *Journal of Acquired Immune Deficiency Syndromes and Human Retrovirology* 10(1):82–89.

Haffner D and Wagoner J. 1999. Vast majority of Americans support sexuality education. *SIECUS Report* 27(6):22–23.

Hammett TM, Gaiter JL, Crawford C. 1998. Reaching seriously at-risk populations: Health interventions in criminal justice settings. *Health Education and Behavior* 25(1):99–120.

Hammett TM, Rhodes W, Harmon P. 1999. HIV/AIDS and other infectious diseases among correctional inmates and releasees: A public health problem and opportunity (Oral Abstract). National HIV Prevention Conference; August 31, 1999; Atlanta.

Harris and Associates. 1988. Sexual material on American network television during the 1987–1988 season. New York: Planned Parenthood Federation of America.

Health Resources and Services Administration. 1995. Progress and Challenges in Linking Incarcerated Individuals with HIV/AIDS to Community Services. Washington, DC: HRSA.

Heimer R. 1998. Can syringe exchange serve as a conduit to substance abuse treatment? *Journal of Substance Abuse Treatment* 15(3):183–191.

Henderson AS. 1988. *An Introduction to Social Psychiatry.* New York: Oxford University Press.

Herek G. 1999. AIDS and stigma. *American Behavioral Scientist* 42(7):1105–1103.

Herek GM and Capitanio JP. 1998. AIDS stigma and HIV-related beliefs in the United States: Results from a national telephone survey (Abstract 44173). XIIth International Conference on AIDS, Jun 28–Jul 3, 1998. Geneva.

Herek GM and Capitanio JP. 1999. AIDS stigma and sexual prejudice. *American Behavioral Scientist* 42(7):1130–1147.

Herek GM and Glunt EK. 1988. An epidemic of stigma. Public reactions to AIDS. *American Psychologist* 43(11):886–891.

Herek G, Mitnick L, Burris S, Chesney M, Devine P, Fullilove M, Fullilove R, Gunther H, Levi J, Michaels S, Novick A, Pryor J, Snyder M, Sweeney T. 1998. Workshop report: AIDS and stigma: A conceptual framework and research agenda. *AIDS and Public Policy Journal* 13(1):36–47.

Horgan C and Hodgkin D. 1999. Mental illness and substance abuse among low-income populations. In Lillie-Blanton M, Martinez R, Lyons B, Rowland D (Eds.), *Access to Health Care: Promises and Prospects for Low-Income Americans.* Washington, DC: Henry J. Kaiser Family Foundation.

Hu DJ, Frey R, Costa SJ, Massey J, Ryan J, Fleming PL, D'Errico S, Ward JW, Buehler J. 1994. Geographical AIDS rates and socio-economic variables in the Newark, New Jersey, metropolitan area. *AIDS and Public Policy* 9(1):20–25.

Hubbard RL, Craddock SG, Flynn PM, Anderson J, Etheridge RM. 1997. Overview of 1-year follow-up outcomes in the Drug Abuse Treatment Outcome Study (DATOS). *Psychology of Addictive Behaviors* 11(4):568–576.

Institute of Medicine. 1990. *Treating Drug Problems: Volume 1.* Gerstein DR and Harwood HJ (Eds.). Washington, DC: National Academy Press.

Institute of Medicine. 1995a. *The Best Intentions: Unintended Pregnancy and the Well-Being of Children and Families.* Brown SS and Eisenberg L (Eds.). Washington, DC: National Academy Press.

Institute of Medicine. 1995b. *Federal Regulation of Methadone Treatment.* Rettig RA and Yarmolinksky A (Eds.). Washington, DC: National Academy Press.

Institute of Medicine. 1997a. *Dispelling the Myths about Addiction: Strategies to Increase Understanding and Strengthen Research.* Washington, DC: National Academy Press.

Institute of Medicine. 1997b. *The Hidden Epidemic: Confronting Sexually Transmitted Diseases.* Eng T and Butler W (Eds.). Washington, DC: National Academy Press.

Institute of Medicine. 1998. *Bridging the Gap Between Practice and Research: Forging Partnerships with Community-Based Drug and Alcohol Treatment.* Lamb S, Greenlick MR, and McCarty D (Eds.). Washington, DC: National Academy Press.

Joint United Nations Programme on HIV/AIDS (UNAIDS). 1998. *Partners in Prevention: International Case Studies of the Effective Health Promotion Practices in HIV/AIDS.* Geneva, Switzerland: UNAIDS.

Joint United Nations Programme on HIV/AIDS (UNAIDS). 1999. *Acting Early to Prevent AIDS: The Case of Senegal.* UNAIDS Best Practices Collection. Geneva, Switzerland: UNAIDS.

Joint United Nations Programme on HIV/AIDS (UNAIDS). 2000. Uganda: Epidemiological Fact Sheet on HIV/AIDS and Sexually Transmitted Infections: 2000 Update. Geneva, Switzerland: UNAIDS.

Kaiser Family Foundation. 1998. Sex in the 90's: Kaiser Family Foundation/ABC television 1998 national survey of Americans on sex and sexual health. Washington, DC.

Kaiser Family Foundation. 1999a. Hearing their Voices: A Qualitative Research Study on HIV Testing and Higher-Risk Teens. Menlo Park, CA .

Kaiser Family Foundation. 1999b. Policy and Politics: Sex Education in Public Secondary Schools. Issue Update. Washington, DC: Kaiser Family Foundation.

Kaiser Family Foundation. 1999c. Welfare Policy and Reproductive Health: Abstinence Unless Married Programs. Issue Brief. Washington, DC: Kaiser Family Foundation.

Kaplan EH. 1995. Probability Models of Needle Exchange. *Operations Research* 43:558–569.

Kaplan EH and O'Keefe E. 1993. Let the needles do the talking! Evaluating the New Haven Needle Exchange. *Interfaces* 23(1):7–26.

Katz MH. 1997. AIDS epidemic in San Francisco among men who report sex with men: Successes and challenges of HIV prevention. *Journal of Acquired Immune Deficiency Syndromes and Human Retrovirology* 14 (Suppl 2):S38–S46.

Kirby D. 2000. School-based interventions to prevent unprotected sex and HIV among adolescents. In Peterson and DiClemente R (Eds.). *Handbook of HIV Prevention* . New York: Kluwer Academy/Plenum Publishers.

Kirby D. 1995. Sex and HIV/AIDS education in schools. *British Medical Journal* 311(7002):403.

Kirby D and Brown N. 1996. School condom availability programs in the United States. *Family Planning Perspectives* 28(5):196–202.

Kleiman MAR. 1992. *Against Excess: Drug Policy for Results*. New York: Basic Books.

Klonoff EA and Landrine H. 1999. Do blacks believe that HIV/AIDS is a government conspiracy against them? *Preventive Medicine* 28(5):451–457.

Kraft MK, Rothbard AB, Hadley TR, McLellan AT, Asch DA. 1997. Are Supplementary Services Provided During Methadone Maintenance Really Cost-Effective? *American Journal of Psychiatry* 154(9):1214–1219.

Landrine H and Klonoff E. 1997. The schedule of racist events: A measure of racial discrimination and a study of its negative physical and mental health consequences. *Journal of Black Psychology* 23:50–7.

Landry DJ, Kaeser L, Richards CL. 1999. Abstinence promotion and the provision of information about contraception in public school district sexuality education policies. *Family Planning Perspectives* 31(6):280–286.

Lehman JS, Hecht FM, Wortley P, Lansky A, Stevens M, Fleming P. Are at-risk populations less concerned about HIV infection in the HAART era? (Abstract 198.) 7th Conference on Retroviruses and Opportunistic Infections; Jan. 30–Feb. 2, 2000. San Francisco, CA.

Lewis JE, Malow RM, Ireland SJ. 1997. HIV/AIDS risk in heterosexual college students. A review of a decade of literature. *Journal of American College Health* 45(4):147–158.

Longshore D, Hseih S, Danila B, Anglin MD. 1993. Drug-related HIV risk and cocaine preference among injection drug users in Los Angeles. *Journal of Drug Education* 23:259–272.

Lowry DT, Shidler JA. 1993. Prime time TV portrayals of sex, "safe sex" and AIDS: A longitudinal analysis. *Journalism Quarterly* 70:628–637.

Lurie P and Drucker E. 1997. An opportunity lost: HIV infections associated with lack of a national needle-exchange programme in the USA. *Lancet* 349(9052):604–608.

Lurie P, Fernandes ME, Hughes V, Arevalo EI, Hudes ES, Reingold A, Hearst N. 1995. Socioeconomic status and risk of HIV-1, syphilis and hepatitis B infection among sex workers in Sao Paulo State, Brazil. Instituto Adolfo Lutz Study Group. *AIDS* 9 (Suppl 1):S31–S37.

Lurie P and Reingold AL (Eds.). 1993. *The Public Health Impact of Needle Exchange Programs in the United States and Abroad: Summary, Conclusions, and Recommendations.* San Francisco: University of California at San Francisco.

Magura S, Rosenblum A, Rodriguez EM. 1998. Changes in HIV risk behaviors among cocaine-using methadone patients. *Journal of Addictive Diseases* 17(4):71–90.

Makadon HJ, Silin JG. 1995. Prevention of HIV infection in primary care: Current practices, future possibilities. *Annals of Internal Medicine* 123(9):715–719.

Marquis J. 2000. Syphilis Outbreak Grows in L.A. *Los Angeles Times*, Metro Section April 8.

Maynard R. 2000. Abstinence-only Education and STDs: Theory, Practice and Evaluation of Programs Funded Under Title V. Presentation made to the Institute of Medicine Committee on HIV Prevention Strategies, March 1, Washington, DC.

Mays VM and Cochran SD. 1988. Issues in the perception of AIDS risk and risk reduction activities by black and Hispanic/Latina women. *American Psychologist* 43(11):949–957.

McKusick D, Mark TL, King E, Harwood R, Buck JA, Dilonardo J, Genuardi JS. 1998. Spending for mental health and substance abuse treatment, 1996. *Health Affairs* 17(5):147–157.

Merrill JM, Laux LF, Thornby JI. 1990. Why doctors have difficulty with sex histories. *Southern Medical Journal* 83(6):613–617.

Metzger DS, Woody GE, McLellan AT, O'Brien CP, Druley P, Navaline H, DePhilippis D, Stolley P, Abrutyn E. 1993. Human immunodeficiency virus seroconversion among intravenous drug users in- and out-of-treatment: An 18-month prospective follow-up. *Journal of Acquired Immune Deficiency Syndromes* 6(9):1049–1056.

Mickler SE. 1993. Perceptions of vulnerability: Impact on AIDS-preventive behavior among college adolescents. *AIDS Education and Prevention* 5(1):43–53.

Mumola C. 1999. Substance abuse and treatment, state and federal prisoners, 1997. Bureau of Justice Statistics Special Report. Washington, DC: U.S. Department of Justice, Office of Justice Programs.

Murphy SL. 2000. *Deaths: Final Data for 1998.* National Vital Statistics Reports. Hyattsville, MD: National Center for Health Statistics.

National Center on Addiction and Substance Abuse at Columbia University (CASA). 1998. *Behind Bars: Substance Abuse and America's Prison Population.* New York City: CASA

National Institute of Justice, Centers for Disease Control and Prevention. 1995. *1994 Update: HIV/AIDS and STDs in Correctional Facilities.* Washington, DC: Department of Justice.

National Institute of Justice, Centers for Disease Control and Prevention, Bureau of Justice Statistics. 1999. *1996–1997 Update: HIV/AIDS, STDs, and TB in Correctional Facilities.* Washington, DC: Department of Justice.

National Institutes of Health. 1997a. Interventions to prevent HIV risk behaviors. *NIH Consensus Statement* 15(2):1–41.

National Institutes of Health. 1997b. Effective Medical Treatment of Opiate Addiction. Consensus Development Conference Statement 108. Bethesda, MD: NIH.

National Research Council. 1989. *AIDS: Sexual Behavior and Intravenous Drug Use.* Turner CF, Miller HG and Moses LE (Eds.). Washington, DC: National Academy Press.

National Research Council, Institute of Medicine. 1993. *The Social Impact of AIDS in the United States.* Jonsen AR, and Stryker J (Eds.). Washington, DC: National Academy Press.

National Research Council, Institute of Medicine. 1995. *Preventing HIV Transmission: The Role of Sterile Needles and Bleach.* Normand J, Vlahov D, and Moses LE (Eds.). Washington, DC: National Academy Press.

Nelson KE, Celentano DD, Eiumtrakol S, Hoover DR, Beyrer C, Suprasert S, Kuntolbutra S, Khamboonruang C. 1996. Changes in sexual behavior and a decline in HIV infection among young men in Thailand. *New England Journal of Medicine* 335(5):297–303.

North American Syringe Exchange Network (NASEN). 2000. Email Communication from J. Rustad, May 17.

Office of National Drug Control Policy (ONDCP). 2000a. Fact Sheet: Methadone [Web Page]. Located at: www.whitehousedrugpolicy.gov/drugfact/factsheet.html.

Office of National Drug Control Policy (ONDCP). 2000b. *FY 2001 Budget Report.* Washington, DC: ONDCP.

Office of National Drug Control Policy (ONDCP). 2000c. *The National Drug Control Strategy: 2000 Annual Report.* Washington, DC: ONDCP.

Office of National Drug Control Policy (ONDCP). 1999. *National Drug Control Strategy, 1999 Annual Report.* Washington, DC: ONDCP.

Office of Technology Assessment (OTA). 1990. *The Effectiveness of Drug Abuse Treatment: Implications for Controlling AIDS/HIV Infection. Background Paper 6.* Washington, DC: OTA.

Pinkerton SD and Abramson PR. 1997. Effectiveness of condoms in preventing HIV transmission. *Social Science and Medicine* 44(9):1303–1312.

Pollack H, Khoshnood K, Altice F. 1999. Health care delivery strategies for criminal offenders. *Journal of Health Care Finance* 26(1):63–77.

Poppen PJ and Reisen CA. 1997. Perception of risk and sexual self-protective behavior: A methodological critique. *AIDS Education and Prevention* 9(4):373–390.

Presidential Advisory Council on HIV/AIDS (PACHA). 2000. PACHA recommendations. Washington, DC: PACHA.

Risen CB. 1995. A guide to taking a sexual history. *Psychiatric Clinics of North America* 18(1):39–53.

Roper Organization. 1991. *AIDS: Public Attitudes and Education Needs.*

Schieman S. 1998. Gender and AIDS-related psychosocial processes: A study of perceived susceptibility, social distance, and homophobia. *AIDS Education and Prevention* 10(3):264–277.

Sexuality Information and Education Council of the United States (SIECUS). 1999. *Between the Lines: States' Implementation of the Federal Government's Section 510 (b) Abstinence Education Program in Fiscal Year 1998.* New York: SIECUS.

Simon PA, Hu DJ, Diaz T, Kerndt PR. 1995. Income and AIDS rates in Los Angeles County. *AIDS* 9(3):281–284.

STD Communication Roundtable. 1996. STDTALK: Spreading the word about sexually transmitted diseases. Washington, DC: Ogilvy, Adams, and Rinehart.

Stolberg SG. 1998. Clinton Decides Not to Finance Needle Program. *The New York Times:*A1, April 21.

Strain EC, Bigelow GE, Liebson IA, Stitzer ML. 1999. Moderate- vs. high-dose methadone in the treatment of opioid dependence: A randomized trial. *Journal of the American Medical Association* 281(11):1000–1005.

Substance Abuse and Mental Health Services Administration (SAMHSA) 2000. *HIV Strategic Plan.* Washington, DC: SAMHSA.

Substance Abuse and Mental Health Services Administration (SAMHSA). 1999a. *Uniform Facility Data Set (UFDS): 1997 Data on Substance Abuse Treatment Facilities.* Washington, DC: SAMHSA.

Substance Abuse and Mental Health Services Administration (SAMHSA). 1999b. New Federal Rules Proposed to Improve Quality and Oversight of Methadone Treatment. Press Release. July 22.

Swartz JA, Lurigio AJ, Goldstein P. 2000. Severe mental illness and substance use disorders among former Supplemental Security Income beneficiaries for drug addiction and alcoholism. *Archives of General Psychiatry* 57(7):701–707.

Thomas SB and Quinn SC. 1991. The Tuskegee Syphilis Study, 1932 to 1972: Implications for HIV education and AIDS risk education programs in the black community. *American Journal of Public Health* 81(11):1498–1505.

Valleroy LA, Weinstein B, Jones TS, Groseclose SL, Rolfs RT, Kassler WJ. 1995. Impact of increased legal access to needles and syringes on community pharmacies' needle and syringe sales—Connecticut, 1992–1993. *Journal of Acquired Immune Deficiency Syndromes and Human Retrovirology* 10(1):73–81.

Walker EA, Katon WJ, Hansom J, Harrop-Griffiths J, Holm L, Jones ML, Hickok L, Jemelka RP. 1992. Medical and psychiatric symptoms in women with childhood sexual abuse. *Psychosomatic Medicine* 54(6):658–664.

Weisner C, McCarty D, Schmidt L. 1999. New directions in alcohol and drug treatment under managed care. *American Journal of Managed Care* 5 (Spec No):SP57–SP69.

Williams LA, Klausner JD, Whittington WL, Handsfield HH, Celum C, Holmes KK. 1999. Elimination and reintroduction of primary and secondary syphilis. *American Journal of Public Health* 89(7):1093–1097.

Zierler S, Krieger N. 1997. Reframing women's risk: Social inequalities and HIV infection. *Annual Review of Public Health* 18:401–436.

Zierler S, Krieger N, Tang Y, Coady W, Siegfried E, DeMaria A, Auerbach J. 2000. Economic deprivation and AIDS incidence in Massachusetts. *American Journal of Public Health* 90(7):1064–1073.

Appendixes

A

The Changing Epidemic

AIDS TRENDS IN THE UNITED STATES[1]

The first cases of AIDS were reported in 1981 (CDC, 1981). Through 1999, a total of 733,374 AIDS cases and 430,411 AIDS-related deaths were reported. Approximately 99 percent (724,656) of AIDS cases were reported among adults and adolescents age 13 and older; 1 percent (8,718) were reported among children under the age of 13. In 1999, 46,400 new AIDS cases were reported (CDC, 2000b). Cases reported in the United States account for less than 1 percent of the estimated cases reported worldwide (Text Box A.1).

During the first decade of the epidemic, the number of new AIDS cases rose by between 65 percent and 90 percent annually (CDC, 1996).[2] In 1996, AIDS incidence[3] and AIDS deaths declined for the first time in the history of the epidemic (CDC, 1997) (Figure A.1). These declines can be attributed to advances in antiretroviral therapies that slow disease

---

[1]This section relies heavily on information contained in "The States of the HIV/AIDS Epidemic" (Kaiser Family Foundation, 2000).

[2]These numbers must be interpreted with caution, however, as the AIDS case definition changed in 1985, 1987, and 1993.

[3]The expansion of the AIDS case definition in 1993 created a temporary distortion in AIDS trend incidence. By the end of 1996, the temporary distortion caused by reporting prevalent and incident cases that met criteria added in 1993 had almost entirely disappeared. Figure A.1 reflects this distortion in the AIDS incidence trend.

TEXT BOX A.1
The Global HIV/AIDS Pandemic

In 1999, an estimated 34.3 million people worldwide were living with HIV or AIDS. Since the beginning of the pandemic, AIDS has resulted in more than 18.8 million deaths, including 2.8 million during 1999 alone. More than 95 percent of all HIV-infected people live in the developing world, and approximately 70 percent of all HIV-infected people live in sub-Saharan Africa (UNAIDS, 2000).

The AIDS epidemic is having devastating effects on the social and economic welfare and health of developing nations. The resulting instability, in addition to the public health implications of increased travel and migration, has direct implications for the United States. The Committee suggests these issues be addressed in a future study focused on optimizing the U.S. role in fighting the global pandemic.

---

progression and extend the lives of people with AIDS, and in part to the success of earlier HIV prevention efforts (CDC, 1999b). Since mid-1998, however, the number of AIDS cases and deaths diagnosed each quarter has remained relatively stable (CDC, 2000d). The Centers for Disease Control and Prevention (CDC) suggests that the stabilization is likely due to a combination of several factors including: treatment failure and the fact that some people have problems adhering to treatment regimens; the fact that HIV prevention efforts have already reached many of those individuals who are most disposed to treatment; and the fact that many people cannot be reached with early testing and treatment (CDC, 2000d).

Between 1993 and 1999, the estimated number of people living with AIDS increased by 69 percent (CDC, 2000b) (Figure A.1). Today, the number of people reported to be living with AIDS[4] (299,944) is at an all-time high (CDC, 2000b).

Modes of Transmission

In the United States, the primary modes of HIV transmission have been sexual intercourse and injection drug use. Of the 724,656 AIDS cases reported among adults and adolescents since the beginning of the epidemic, 47 percent have been linked to sex between men, 25 percent to injection drug use, 10 percent to heterosexual intercourse, 6 percent to men who have sex with men and inject drugs, and 2 percent to contaminated blood or blood products (CDC, 2000b). In recent years, however, disease patterns have begun to shift. A declining proportion of new AIDS cases now is being attributed to sex between men, and an increasing proportion of cases is being linked to heterosexual exposure. However, MSM remains the single largest exposure group (CDC, 2000b). The pro-

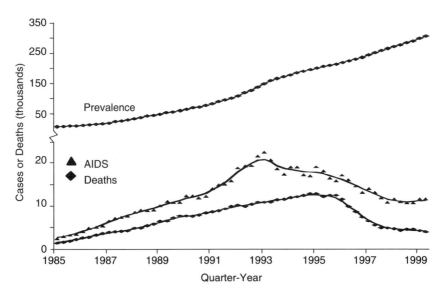

FIGURE A.1 Estimated AIDS incidence, deaths, and prevalence in adults, quarter-year of diagnosis or death, 1985–1999, United States. SOURCE: CDC, 2000c.

portion of AIDS cases linked to sex between men declined from approximately 65 percent in 1985 to 40 percent in 1998 (CDC, 2000b; CDC, 2000c) (Figure A.2). In contrast, the proportion of AIDS cases linked to heterosexual transmission accounted for less than 5 percent in 1985 but increased to 15 percent in 1999. The proportion of cases linked to injection drug use rose through the early 1990s, but has declined in recent years. Injection drug use accounted for 22 percent of new AIDS cases in 1999 (CDC, 2000b).[4]

Perinatal transmission is the primary route of HIV infection among children under 13 years of age. With the exception of children infected through transfusions and blood products, which occurred mostly in the early 1980s, the vast majority of children with AIDS (92 percent) were infected in the course of pregnancy, delivery, or breast feeding (IOM, 1999). In the early 1990s, roughly 1,000 children were diagnosed with

---

[4]Since the surveillance system is hierarchical, any admission by an HIV-infected person of injection drug use after 1977 will result in assignment to that risk exposure category, even if a given individual might be much more likely to have acquired HIV through heterosexual routes. Furthermore, the "no identified risk" persons are often reassigned to the heterosexual risk exposure category if resources are applied for re-interviews. Thus, this hierarchical scheme could minimize the magnitude of the heterosexual epidemic.

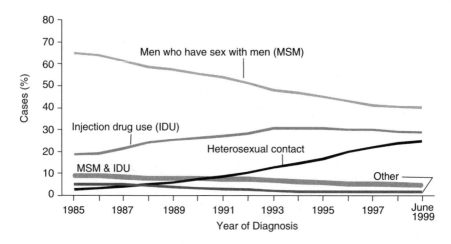

FIGURE A.2 Adult/adolescent AIDS cases by exposure category and year of diagnosis, 1985–June 1999. SOURCE: CDC, 2000c.

AIDS each year (Figure A.3). One of the greatest successes in HIV prevention occurred with the 1994 finding that administration of the antiretroviral drug zidovudine during pregnancy and childbirth could reduce the chances of perinatal transmission by two-thirds (Connor et al., 1994). The rapid implementation and use of zidovudine and other antiretroviral drugs in clinical settings, combined with efforts to identify and treat HIV-infected pregnant women through HIV screening in prenatal care settings, led to dramatic declines in the number of pediatric AIDS cases (Figure A.3). Between 1993 and 1999, the number of pediatric AIDS cases declined by 75 percent (CDC, 2000b).

The Changing Demographic Face of the Epidemic

The demographic populations affected by the epidemic have evolved over time. During the 1990s, women, youth, and racial and ethnic minorities accounted for a growing proportion of new AIDS cases. Geographic distributions have also shifted, with a growing proportion of cases emerging in rural and smaller urban areas.

AIDS Cases in Women

The increases in AIDS cases among women is consistent with the increase of cases linked to heterosexual transmission. The proportion of annual new AIDS cases among women tripled, from 7 percent to 23 per-

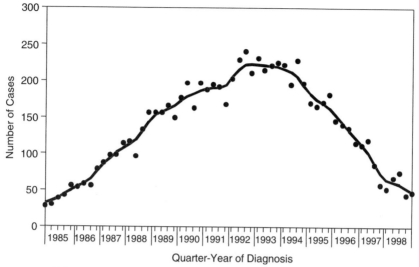

FIGURE A.3 Perinatally acquired AIDS cases by quarter-year of diagnosis, 1985–1998, United States. SOURCE: CDC, 2000e.

cent, between 1986 and 1999 (Kaiser Family Foundation, 2000). Women now comprise 17 percent of the total AIDS cases reported since 1981, and 20 percent of the population living with AIDS (CDC, 2000b).

Women in racial and ethnic minority groups have been disproportionately affected by the epidemic. In 1999, 81 percent of new AIDS cases among women were reported among Hispanic and African-American women. These women represented 23 percent of the U.S. population of women (U.S. Census Bureau, 1999). The AIDS case rate among African-American women (49.0 per 100,000) was more than 20 times the rate among Caucasian women (2.3 per 100,000), while the rate among Hispanic women (14.9 per 100,000) was more than six times the rate among Caucasian women (CDC, 2000b).

AIDS Cases in Youth

AIDS has had a major impact on teenagers and young adults. In 1998, AIDS was the ninth leading cause of death among youth ages 15–24, and the fifth leading cause of death among individuals 25–44, many of whom were infected as teenagers (Murphy, 2000). Young women, and particularly members of racial and ethnic minorities have been disproportionately affected. In 1999, females accounted for 58 percent of reported AIDS cases among 13- to 19-year-olds and 38 percent of cases among 20- to 24-year-olds. Almost half of the new AIDS cases in the 13–24 age group (43 percent) were among African Americans, and almost one-quarter (21 percent) were among Hispanics (CDC, 2000b).

Sexual exposure is the primary route of infection among young people. Most young men are infected through sex with other men, while most young women are infected through heterosexual exposure. In 1999, 50 percent of AIDS cases among males ages 13–24 were acquired through sex with other men, and 8 percent through sex with women. In the same year, nearly half of new AIDS cases (47 percent) among females ages 13–24 were acquired heterosexually. Furthermore, a proportion of "risk not specified" cases would fall into these risk exposure categories if the data were available (CDC, 2000b).[5]

AIDS Cases in Racial and Ethnic Minorities

Racial and ethnic minorities, particularly African Americans and Hispanics, have been disproportionately affected by the AIDS epidemic. The proportion of new cases among African Americans and Hispanics has increased over time, while the proportion of AIDS cases among Caucasians has decreased. Since 1996, African Americans have accounted for a greater proportion of AIDS cases than Caucasians. The proportion of cases has remained relatively stable in American Indians and Asian/Pacific Islanders. These two groups comprise approximately one percent of all AIDS cases (CDC, 2000b; CDC, 2000a) (Figure A.4).

Although African Americans and Hispanics, taken together, accounted for 66 percent of all new AIDS cases in 1999 (CDC, 2000b), these groups comprised only an estimated 23 percent of the total U.S. population (CDC, 2000a). In 1999, the AIDS case rate[6] among African Americans (66.0 per 100,000) was more than eight times the rate among Caucasians (7.6 per 100,000), while the AIDS case rate among Hispanics (25.6 per 100,000) was three times higher than for Caucasians (CDC, 2000b).

While the number of AIDS-related deaths has declined[7] among all racial and ethnic groups, the decline has been slower among African Americans and Hispanics. AIDS remains the leading cause of death among African Americans between the ages of 25 and 44, and the third

---

[5]Nearly half of all AIDS cases did not have a risk reported or identified.

[6]The AIDS case rate includes both adult and pediatric cases.

[7]Recent data suggest the declining trends in AIDS deaths and cases have stabilized (CDC, 2000d).

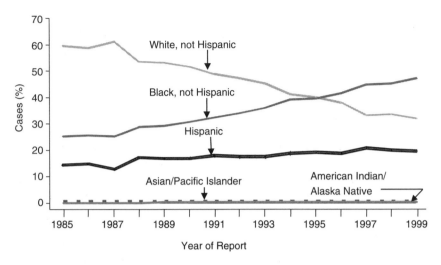

FIGURE A.4 Proportion of AIDS cases, by race/ethnicity and year of report, 1985–1999. SOURCE: CDC, 2000a.

leading cause of death among Hispanics in this age group. Among Caucasians of the same age group, AIDS is the fifth leading cause of death (Murphy, 2000). In 1998, the most recent year for which data are available, the death rate from AIDS for African Americans (32.5 per 100,000) was nearly 10 times the rate among Caucasians (3.3 per 100,000) (Gayle, 2000).

Geographic Distribution of AIDS Cases

AIDS cases have been reported in all 50 states, the District of Columbia, and the U.S. territories. Ten states and territories account for almost three-quarters (72 percent) of all AIDS cases.[8] Four states—New York, California, Florida, and Texas—represent 52 percent of cumulative AIDS cases and 47 percent of new AIDS cases reported in 1999, yet these states contain only 32 percent of the U.S. population (CDC, 2000b; U.S. Census Bureau, 1999). In 1999, the states and territories with the highest AIDS incidence rate 100,000 population were the District of Columbia (161.5 cases per 100,000 population), New York (42.3 cases per 100,000 population), Florida (36.2 cases per 100,000 population), Puerto Rico (32.1 cases

---

[8]The 10 states and territories with the highest total number of AIDS cases include: New York, California, Florida, Texas, New Jersey, Puerto Rico, Illinois, Pennsylvania, Georgia, and Maryland.

per 100,000 population), and Maryland (29.5 cases per 100,000 population) (see Figure A.5). These figures compare with the national AIDS incidence rate in 1999 of 16.7 cases per 100,000 population (CDC, 2000b).

Historically, AIDS cases have been largely concentrated in urban areas. In 1999, 79 percent of AIDS cases were diagnosed in metropolitan areas with populations of 500,000 or more. Ten metropolitan areas (New York City, Los Angeles, San Francisco, Miami, Washington, D.C., Chicago, Houston, Philadelphia, Newark, and Atlanta) accounted for almost half of the cumulative reported AIDS cases. In terms of new AIDS cases per 100,000 persons, the most heavily affected metropolitan areas in 1999 were New York City (72.7 per 100,000), Miami/Ft. Lauderdale (65.3 and 61.2 per 100,000, respectively), Columbia, S.C. (54.6 per 100,000), and San Francisco (50.8 per 100,000) (CDC, 2000b).

While the U.S. epidemic has been perceived largely as an urban phenomenon, AIDS cases in rural areas have been among the most rapidly rising subset of the new cases reported to the CDC. The fastest growing rural epidemic is in the South, followed by the Northeast, the West, and the Midwest. As a proportion of the total cases, heterosexual transmission is more common in small town/rural settings than in urban sites; women and racial and ethnic minorities represent a substantial subset of nonurban cases (Wortley and Fleming, 1997; Graham et al., 1995).

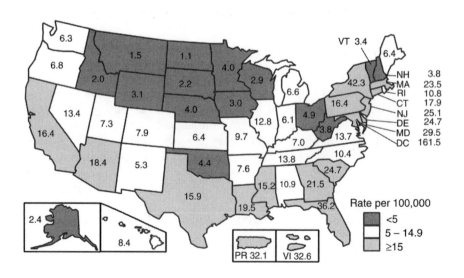

FIGURE A.5 AIDS case rates per 100,000 population, reported in 1999 (CDC, 2000c).

AIDS and Co-Occurring Conditions

AIDS is often part of an overlapping cluster of epidemics. AIDS cases are increasingly concentrated in disadvantaged populations that have high rates of poverty, homelessness, unemployment, and inadequate access to health care. AIDS also overlaps with other illnesses, including drug addiction, mental disorders, sexually transmitted diseases (STDs), tuberculosis (TB), and hepatitis. These conditions may contribute to the risk of HIV exposure and transmission and may complicate HIV prevention and therapeutic efforts.

AIDS has had a disproportionate impact on the poor and disadvantaged populations. Over the course of the epidemic, there has been a steady increase in the numbers of HIV-infected persons who are homeless and marginally housed (Bangsberg et al., 2000; Zolopa et al., 1994). Many of these individuals lack access to necessary health services, including primary medical care, substance abuse treatment, and HIV care (including treatment with new antiretroviral therapies) (Acuff et al., 1999). Recent studies suggest that poverty contributes to HIV infection risk in several ways. Socioeconomic instability may contribute to higher rates of prostitution, drug use, incarceration, and family disruption, all of which are linked to the spread of HIV (Fournier and Carmichael, 1998).

The link between substance abuse and risk of HIV infection is well-established (IOM, 1997; NRC and IOM, 1995; NRC, 1989). Injection drug users are primarily infected through sharing of contaminated injection equipment, which acts as a vector for HIV-infected blood (NRC and IOM, 1995). HIV infection among injection drug users also poses a threat to their sexual partners and children (NRC and IOM, 1995). Use of non-injection drugs (e.g., alcohol, crack cocaine, methamphetamines, and inhalants) also can impair decision-making, thereby increasing the likelihood of HIV transmission and infection through high-risk behaviors (e.g., unprotected sex or trading sex for drugs) (IOM, 1997). Immunosuppression caused by long-term use of alcohol and drugs increases the likelihood of infection and, among infected persons, increases the development of AIDS-related opportunistic illnesses (Acuff et al., 2000).

Mental illness also can increase HIV infection and transmission risk (Diamond and Buskin, 2000; Marks et al., 1998). Although some mental disorders may exist prior to the HIV diagnosis (e.g., depression and personality disorders), others may develop during the course of the disease (e.g., HIV-associated dementia). Serious mental illness increases the likelihood of high-risk sexual behaviors or substance abuse, and thus may contribute to treatment nonadherence. Individuals with severe and persistent mental illness (e.g., schizophrenia) often experience high rates of unemployment, poverty, and homelessness, which can increase the complexity associated with preventing and treating their HIV disease (Rabkin and Chesney, 1999; Susser et al., 1995; Susser et al., 1997a; Susser et al., 1997b).

The presence of sexually transmitted diseases may increase both susceptibility to HIV infection and the infectiousness of people who already have HIV. Epidemiological studies suggest that people may be two to five times more likely to become HIV-infected when other STDs are present (Levine et al., 1998; Patterson et al., 1998; IOM, 1997). Similarly, studies suggest that for HIV-infected individuals, the presence of another STD infection increases the likelihood of transmitting HIV to sexual partners (e.g., through genital lesions or increased concentration of HIV in genital secretions) (Cohen et al., 1997; CDC, 1998a).

HIV also overlaps with the spread of other diseases, including TB and hepatitis B and C. Because HIV infection suppresses the body's immune system, HIV-infected persons are at increased risk of developing TB and, if infected, are 100 times more likely to progress to active TB than those not infected with HIV. The CDC estimates that 10 to 15 percent of all TB cases, and 30 percent of cases among individuals age 25 to 44, occur among HIV-infected individuals (CDC, 1998b). Moreover, a recent study found that common HIV and TB treatments may be incompatible (Spradling, 2000). In addition, because HIV-infection accelerates the progression of liver disease and cirrhosis that hepatitis C causes, co-infected individuals may have limited tolerance for antiretroviral therapy, as many of the drugs have hepatic side effects (Ostrow, 1999).

HIV INCIDENCE AND PREVALENCE

In contrast to the epidemiology of AIDS, less is known about either the incidence and prevalence of HIV, or about the geographical, racial, or age distribution of infections. Estimates of HIV incidence and prevalence can be derived from a number of sources, although none provide a complete or accurate picture of true HIV incidence or prevalence. First, statistical estimates can be made by reverse calculations ("back calculations") from reported AIDS cases, incorporating established patterns of disease progression (Brookmeyer and Gail, 1994). Recent developments in therapy for HIV and AIDS have at least temporally decoupled HIV infection and its progression to AIDS (Hammer et al., 1996; Collier et al., 1996). As a result, the timing of the progression from HIV infection to AIDS and from AIDS to death is increasingly difficult to predict, making HIV incidence and prevalence estimates based on AIDS cases much less accurate (CDC, 1999a). Estimates can also be derived from the growing number of states that have made HIV a reportable disease (CDC, 1999a). The accuracy of these data is limited, however, due to biases in the reported data (i.e., only individuals who seek or are offered testing are reflected) (See Chapter 2). The distribution of HIV incidence and prevalence (e.g., by risk groups, race, geography, or age) can also be derived from ongoing cohort studies (e.g., the Multicenter AIDS Cohort Study of gay men) (Kaslow et al., 1987). Finally, estimates can be derived from CDC's family of seroprevalence surveys, including: (1) screening results of blood samples derived from programs testing special populations (e.g., blood donors and applicants to military service and Job Corps), and (2) testing of anonymous blood specimens from smaller studies (e.g., from STD clinics, drug treatment centers, adolescent medical clinics) (Pappaioanou et al., 1990). However, because these studies rely on convenience samples, they cannot be used to produce population-based estimates of HIV incidence and prevalence.

None of these methods or sources of data, however, provides complete and accurate population-based estimates of HIV incidence and prevalence, or of the demographic and geographic distribution of these figures. As discussed in Chapter 2, a new surveillance system, focused on HIV incidence, is needed in order to more effectively guide prevention planning, resource allocation, and evaluation decisions at the national, state, and local levels.

REFERENCES

Acuff C, Archambeault J, Greenberg B, Hoeltzel J, McDaniel JS, Meyer P, Packer C, Parga FJ, Pillen, MB, Rondhovde A, Saldarriaga M, Smith MJ, Stoff D, Wagner D. 1999. *Mental Health Care for People Living with or Affected by HIV/AIDS: A Practical Guide.* Research Triangle Park, NC: Research Triangle Institute.

Bangsberg DR, Hecht FM, Charlebois ED, Zolopa AR, Holodniy M, Sheiner L, Bamberger JD, Chesney MA, Moss A. 2000. Adherence to protease inhibitors, HIV-1 viral load, and development of drug resistance in an indigent population. *AIDS* 14(4):357–366.

Brookmeyer R and Gail MH. 1994. *AIDS Epidemiology: A Quantitative Approach.* New York: Oxford University Press.

Centers for Disease Control and Prevention (CDC). 2000a. HIV/AIDS Surveillance by Race/Ethnicity. Slide sets available on the web: www.cdc.gov/hiv/graphics/minority.htm.

Centers for Disease Control and Prevention (CDC). 2000b. HIV/AIDS Surveillance Report, 1999 11(2).

Centers for Disease Control and Prevention (CDC). 2000c. HIV/AIDS Surveillance—General Epidemiology. Slide sets available on the web: www.cdc.gov/hiv/graphics/surveill.htm.

Centers for Disease Control and Prevention (CDC). 2000d. U.S. AIDS Cases, Deaths, and HIV Infections Appear Stable. AMA Press Briefing, July 8.

Centers for Disease Control and Prevention (CDC). 2000e. HIV/AIDS Surveillance—Perinatal. Slide sets available on the web: www.cdc.gov/hiv/graphics/perinatal.htm.

Centers for Disease Control and Prevention (CDC). 1999a. Guidelines for national human immunodeficiency virus case surveillance, including monitoring for human immunodeficiency virus infection and acquired immunodeficiency syndrome. Centers for Disease Control and Prevention. *Morbidity and Mortality Weekly Report* 48(RR-13):1–31.

Centers for Disease Control and Prevention (CDC). 1999b. HIV/AIDS Surveillance Report, Mid-year 1999:11(1).

Centers for Disease Control and Prevention (CDC). 1998a. HIV prevention through early detection and treatment of other sexually transmitted diseases—United States. *Morbidity and Mortality Weekly Report* 47(RR–12):1–24.

Centers for Disease Control and Prevention (CDC) 1998b. Prevention and treatment of tuberculosis among patients infected with human immunodeficiency virus: Principles of therapy and revised recommendations. *Morbidity and Mortality Weekly Report* 47(RR–20).

Centers for Disease Control and Prevention (CDC). 1997. Update: trends in AIDS incidence—United States, 1996. *Morbidity and Mortality Weekly Report* 46:861–867.

Centers for Disease Control and Prevention (CDC). 1996. 1996 HIV/AIDS Trends Provide Evidence of Success in HIV Prevention and Treatment. Press Release, June.

Centers for Disease Control and Prevention (CDC). 1981. Pneumocystis pneumonia—Los Angeles. *Morbidity and Mortality Weekly Report* 30(21):250–252.

Cohen MS, Hoffman IF, Royce RA, Kazembe P, Dyer JR, Daly CC, Zimba D, Vernazza PL, Maida M, Fiscus SA, Eron J, Jr. 1997. Reduction of concentration of HIV-1 in semen after treatment of urethritis: implications for prevention of sexual transmission of HIV-1. AIDSCAP Malawi Research Group. *Lancet* 349:1868–1873.

Collier AC, Coombs RW, Schoenfeld DA, Bassett RL, Timpone J, Baruch A, Jones M, Facey K, Whitacre C, McAuliffe VJ, Friedman HM, Merigan TC, Reichman RC, Hooper C, Corey L. 1996. Treatment of human immunodeficiency virus infection with saquinavir, zidovudine, and zalcitabine. AIDS Clinical Trials Group. *New England Journal of Medicine* 334(16):1011–1017.

Connor EM, Sperling RS, Gelber R, Kiselev P, Scott G, O'Sullivan MJ, VanDyke R, Bey M, Shearer W, Jacobson RL, Jimenez E, O'Neill E, Bazin B, Delfraissy JF, Culnane M, Coombs R, Elkins M, Moye J, Stratton P, Balsley J. 1994. Reduction of maternal–infant transmission of human immunodeficiency virus type 1 with zidovudine treatment. Pediatric AIDS Clinical Trials Group Protocol 076 Study Group. *New England Journal of Medicine* 331(18):1173–1180.

Diamond C, Buskin S. 2000. Continued risky behavior in HIV-infected youth. *American Journal of Public Health* 90:115–118.

Fournier AM, Carmichael C. 1998. Socioeconomic influences on the transmission of human immunodeficiency virus infection: the hidden risk. *Archives of Family Medicine* 7:214–217.

Gayle HD. 2000. The State of the HIV/AIDS Epidemic. Congressional Staff Briefing. Washington, DC, April 3.

Graham RP, Forrester ML, Wysong JA, Rosenthal TC, James PA. 1995. HIV/AIDS in the rural United States: Epidemiology and health services delivery. *Medical Care Research and Review* 52(4):435–452.

Hammer SM, Katzenstein DA, Hughes MD, Gundacker H, Schooley RT, Haubrich RH, Henry WK, Lederman MM, Phair JP, Niu M, Hirsch MS, Merigan TC. 1996. A trial comparing nucleoside monotherapy with combination therapy in HIV-infected adults with CD4 cell counts from 200 to 500 per cubic millimeter. AIDS Clinical Trials Group Study 175 Study Team. *New England Journal of Medicine* 335(15):1081–1090.

Institute of Medicine. 1997. *The Hidden Epidemic: Confronting Sexually Transmitted Diseases.* Eng T and Butler W (Eds.). Washington, DC: National Academy Press.

Institute of Medicine. 1999. *Reducing the Odds: Preventing Perinatal Transmission of HIV in the United States.* Stoto MA, Almario DA, and McCormick MC (Eds.). Washington, DC: National Academy Press.

Joint United Nations Programme on HIV/AIDS (UNAIDS). June 2000. *Report on the Global HIV/AIDS Epidemic.* New York: United Nations

Kaiser Family Foundation. 2000. The State of the HIV/AIDS Epidemic. Capitol Hill Briefing Series on HIV/AIDS.

Kaslow RA, Ostrow DG, Detels R, Phair JP, Polk BF, Rinaldo CR Jr. 1987. The Multicenter AIDS Cohort Study: Rationale, organization, and selected characteristics of the participants. *American Journal of Epidemiology* 126(2):310–318.

Levine WC, Pope V, Bhoomkar A, Tambe P, Lewis JS, Zaidi AA, Farshy CE, Mitchell S, Talkington DF. 1998. Increase in endocervical CD4 lymphocytes among women with nonulcerative sexually transmitted diseases. *Journal of Infectious Diseases* 177:167–174.

Marks G, Bingman C, Duval TS. 1998. Negative affects and unsafe sex in HIV-positive men. *AIDS and Behavior* 2(2):89–99.

Murphy SL. 2000. *Deaths: Final Data for 1998.* National Vital Statistics Reports. Hyattsville, MD: National Center for Health Statistics.

National Research Council. 1989. *AIDS: Sexual Behavior and Intravenous Drug Use.* Turner CF, Miller HG, and Moses LE (Eds.). Washington, DC: National Academy Press.

National Research Council, Institute of Medicine. 1995. *Preventing HIV Transmission: The Role of Sterile Needles and Bleach.* Normand J, Vlahov D, and Moses LE (Eds.). Washington, DC: National Academy Press.

Ostrow D. 1999. Practical prevention issues. In Ostrow D and Kalichman S (Eds.). *Psychosocial and Public Health Impacts of New HIV Therapies.* New York: Kluwer Academic/Plenum Publishers.

Pappaioanou M, Dondero TJ Jr, Petersen LR, Onorato IM, Sanchez CD, Curran JW. 1990. The family of HIV seroprevalence surveys: Objectives, methods, and uses of sentinel surveillance for HIV in the United States. *Public Health Reports.* 105(2):113–119.

Patterson BK, Landay A, Andersson J, Brown C, Behbahani H, Jiyamapa D, Burki Z, Stanislawski D, Czerniewski MA, Garcia P. 1998. Repertoire of chemokine receptor expression in the female genital tract: Implications for human immunodeficiency virus transmission. *American Journal of Pathology* 153(2):481–490.

Rabkin JG and Chesney MA. 1999. Treatment adherence to HIV medications: The Achilles heel of new therapeutics. In Ostrow D and Kalichman S (Eds.). *Psychosocial and Public Health Impacts of New HIV Therapies.* New York: Kluwer Academic/Plenum Publishers.

Spradling P. 2000. Concurrent use of rifabutin and HAART: Evidence for reduced efficacy? (Abstract TUOR B8277). XIII International AIDS Conference. July 9–14, 2000, Durban, South Africa.

Susser E, Betne P, Valencia E, Goldfinger SM, Lehman AF. 1997a. Injection drug use among homeless adults with severe mental illness. *American Journal of Public Health* 87(5):854–856.

Susser E, Colson P, Jandorf L, Berkman A, Lavelle J, Fennig S, Waniek C, Bromet E. 1997b. HIV infection among young adults with psychotic disorders. *American Journal of Psychiatry* 154(6):864–866.

Susser E, Valencia E, Miller M, Tsai WY, Meyer-Bahlburg H, Conover S. 1995. Sexual behavior of homeless mentally ill men at risk for HIV. *American Journal of Psychiatry* 152(4):583–587.

U.S. Census Bureau. Statistical Abstract of the United States: 1999 (119th edition). Washington, DC: U.S. Census Bureau.

Wortley PM, Fleming PL. 1997. AIDS in women in the United States: Recent trends. *Journal of the American Medical Association* 278:911–916.

Zolopa AR, Hahn JA, Gorter R, Miranda J, Wlodarczyk D, Peterson J, Pilote L, Moss AR. 1994. HIV and tuberculosis infection in San Francisco's homeless adults. Prevalence and risk factors in a representative sample. *Journal of the American Medical Association* 272:455–461.

B

The Prevention Portfolio: Interventions to Prevent HIV Infection

After approximately two decades of research on interventions to prevent HIV infection, there is a wealth of data documenting the results of HIV prevention efforts. The majority of existing prevention strategies are behavioral interventions that try to change sexual and substance use practices that increase risk of exposure to and infection with the virus. There also are interventions that occur on the biomedical or technological level. These have the same goal of preventing new HIV infections, but make use of the advances in clinical medicine, HIV treatment, and biotechnology to lower individuals' susceptibility to HIV infection. In addition, prevention efforts benefit from the treatment of other co-occurring diseases, such as sexually transmitted diseases (STDs), substance abuse, and mental disorders. Still other prevention interventions are societal in that they strive to change the social and environmental factors—such as policies, access to prevention services, and social norms—that contribute to individuals' HIV risk.

All of these types of interventions, in essence, comprise a menu of options that can be used to prevent new HIV infections. Table B.1 presents a summary of the interventions currently available for HIV prevention. The following discussion of these strategies relies on reviews and meta-analyses of the behavioral and biomedical research literature, particularly the Centers for Disease Control and Prevention's Compendium of HIV Prevention Interventions with Evidence of Effectiveness (1999) and the National Institutes of Health Consensus Statement (1997).

TABLE B.1 Biomedical and Behavioral Intervention Strategies Used to Prevent New HIV Infections

Type of Intervention	Populations/ Risk Groups	Outcomes Affected
Behavioral Interventions		
Voluntary counseling and testing	General population	• Decreased HIV risk behavior
Prevention case management	HIV-infected persons, uninfected individuals at elevated risk	• Decreased sexual risk behavior • Decreased drug use-related risk behavior • Increased condom use
Health education and risk reduction counseling (HERR)		
• For adolescents/youth	Adolescents, youth, young people at elevated risk (e.g., homeless, runaway)	• Increased HIV knowledge • Increased positive attitudes toward risk reduction • Decreased sexual risk behavior • Increased condom use • Decreased drug use-related risk behavior
• For injection drug users (IDUs)	IDU	• Decreased sexual risk behavior • Decreased drug-related risk behavior • Increased condom use
• For STD clinic attenders	STD clinic attenders, high-risk adults	• Decreased sexual risk behavior • Increased condom use • Decreased STD incidence • Decreased drug use-related risk behavior
• For men who have sex with men (MSM)	Gay and bisexual men	• Decreased sexual risk behavior • Increased condom use • Decreased drug use-related risk behavior
• For women	Women at elevated risk of infection (including sexual partners of high-risk individuals, such as IDU)	• Increased HIV knowledge • Increased condom use • Decreased sexual risk behavior • Decreased drug use-related risk behavior

Table continued on next page

TABLE B.1 Continued

Type of Intervention	Populations/ Risk Groups	Outcomes Affected
Street/community outreach	High-risk persons, e.g., IDU, CSW, homeless/ runaway youth	• Decreased sexual risk behavior • Decreased drug use-related risk behavior • Increased condom use
School-based HERR education	Adolescents, youth in educational settings (who may or may not be sexually active)	• Increased HIV knowledge • Increased positive attitudes toward risk reduction • Decreased sexual risk behavior • Increased condom use
Prison-based HERR education	Prison inmates	While incarcerated: • Increased HIV knowledge • Increased positive attitudes toward risk reduction When released: • Decreased sexual risk behavior • Increased condom use • Decreased drug use-related risk behavior

Interventions Associated with Treatment of Co-Occurring Conditions

Treatment of sexually transmitted diseases (STD)	Persons with STD infection	• Decreased sexual risk behavior • Decreased susceptibility to HIV due to STD infection
Substance abuse treatment	IDU and other alcohol/ substance abusers	• Decreased number of potential sexual or drug use-related exposures to HIV caused by addiction behavior
Psychiatric/mental health treatment	Persons with psychological disorders or severe mental illness	• Decreased number of potential sexual or drug-use related exposures to HIV caused by psychiatric disorders

Biomedical and Technological Interventions

Administration of zidovudine (AZT) for perinatal transmission	Pregnant HIV-infected women	• Decreased vertical transmission of HIV from mother to infant

TABLE B.1 Continued

Type of Intervention	Populations/ Risk Groups	Outcomes Affected
Postexposure prophylaxis (PEP) for occupational HIV exposure	Health care workers	• Decreased number of new HIV infections caused by work-related exposure to contaminated blood
Postexposure prophylaxis (PEP) for nonoccupational HIV exposure	Persons with sexual or other nonoccupational exposure to HIV	• Unproven efficacy in preventing HIV infection
Screening of blood (and blood products) for HIV	All blood products	• Decreased number of new HIV infections caused by receipt of contaminated blood or blood products
Antiretroviral therapy (ART)	HIV-infected persons	• Decreased infectiousness of HIV-infected person, possibly resulting in decreased sexual transmission of HIV to uninfected sex partners
Societal Interventions Mass media	General population	• Increased HIV/AIDS knowledge • Increased positive attitudes toward risk reduction
Condom social marketing/ availability	General population	• Decreased sexual risk behavior • Increased condom use
Structural (policy, legal) interventions	General population	• Increased access to prevention services and tools (e.g., sterile injection equipment)

BEHAVIORAL INTERVENTIONS

There is an impressive body of evidence for the efficacy of prevention. Behavioral interventions have been shown to be capable of changing risk behaviors related to both sexual practices and substance use in populations of men who have sex with men (ACDP Research Group, 1999; Kegeles et al., 1996; Kelly et al., 1992; Valdiserri et al., 1989), injection drug users (e.g., review by Booth and Watters, 1994), young people (Jemmott et al., 1998; Rotheram-Borus et al., 1997; Stanton et al., 1996; St. Lawrence et al., 1995; Jemmott et al., 1992); heterosexual men (reviewed in Exner et al.,

1999), and women (Sikkema et al., 2000; Exner et al., 1997; DiClemente and Wingood, 1995) . Because behavioral interventions can be tailored to meet the prevention needs and respect the cultural diversity of different populations, they can be adapted for delivery in community settings, including specific venues (e.g., housing developments, STD clinics, schools, and prisons) where at-risk populations are located or come together (e.g., Sikkema et al., 2000; Kamb et al., 1998; NIMH Multisite HIV Prevention Trial Group, 1998; Boyer et al., 1997; Magura et al., 1994; Main et al., 1994; Cohen et al., 1991).

INTERVENTIONS ASSOCIATED WITH THE TREATMENT OF CO-OCCURRING CONDITIONS

Because of the epidemiological synergy between HIV/AIDS and substance abuse, mental health disorders, and STDs, it is crucial to acknowledge the benefit that treatment of these co-occurring conditions can have on the prevention of new HIV infections. There is a wealth of evidence showing that treatment of STDs can reduce individuals' susceptibility to HIV infection, as well as reduce transmission of HIV (CDC, 1998). Further, behavioral counseling by providers during STD treatment can help to encourage risk-reducing behavior change (Cohen, 1995).

Similarly, there is ample evidence that treating substance abuse disorders not only facilitates successful recovery from addiction, but is also associated with reduced HIV infections caused by substance use-related behavior (e.g., sharing injection equipment or engaging in high-risk sexual practices) (Iguchi, 1998; Shoptaw et al., 1998; Moss et al., 1994). Additionally, given that psychiatric disorders and mood disturbances have been shown to be associated with high-risk sexual behavior (Marks et al., 1998; Folkman et al., 1992) and substance use (Drake and Osher, 1997; Regier et al., 1993), treatment for these disorders can lead to reductions in HIV risk behavior. Further, given that mental illness among HIV-infected persons can contribute to poor adherence to antiretroviral therapy (Murphy et al., 1999; Cheever et al., 1998; Schulz et al., 1998), treatment of psychiatric comorbidity could improve medical adherence to antiretroviral treatments and lead to subsequent decreases in viral load and infectiousness.

BIOMEDICAL AND TECHNOLOGICAL INTERVENTIONS

Recent advances in antiretroviral therapies (ARTs) have resulted in the development of several highly effective protocols that can be used for prevention of HIV infection. For example, there is strong evidence that the administration of zidovudine or nevirapine to pregnant HIV-infected women greatly reduces the risk of perinatal transmission of HIV (IOM,

1999; Connor et al., 1994). Similarly, recent evidence suggests that treating HIV-infected persons with low or undetectable viral load have reduced infectiousness to seronegative sexual partners (Quinn et al., 2000). Much more evidence is needed, however, to confirm these findings. Antiretroviral therapy has also been shown to be effective (and is recommended) for reducing the likelihood of infection after occupational exposures (e.g., needle sticks) to HIV (CDC, 1996). Using such treatment may be effective for preventing infection from nonoccupational (e.g., sexual) exposure to HIV, although no data currently exist regarding the effectiveness of this intervention (CDC, 1998). Additionally, the development of sensitive HIV antibody screening assays have been shown to be highly effective in ensuring a blood supply that is virtually free of HIV infection risk (IOM, 1995).

SOCIETAL INTERVENTIONS

Societal prevention interventions show remarkable efficacy in preventing new HIV infections. Such approaches can be highly cost-effective because they can inexpensively reach large numbers of at-risk individuals (Holtgrave et al., 1998; Pinkerton and Holtgrave, 1998). The social marketing of condoms is an example of a societal intervention that has been proven effective for HIV prevention, particularly in developing countries (Ford et al., 1996; Bhave et al., 1995; Ford and Norris, 1993; Ngugi et al., 1988). Condom social marketing seeks to increase the popularity of condoms using advertising and mass media, as well as to increase access to condoms by making them widely available to the general public through community health facilities, promotional events, and other mechanisms (Andreasen, 1995). With combined increases in condom advertising and availability, these campaigns promote the idea that condom use is an attractive, positive behavior, all the while reducing the barriers to engaging in this behavior. Typically, condom social marketing results in increased rates of community level condom use, thereby providing benefit to the multiple goals of HIV and STD prevention.

A nationwide condom advertising and availability program has never occurred in the United States (Bedimo et al., in review). However, smaller-scale studies of condom social marketing in selected areas show such programs are met with great receptivity by individuals, can be very cost effective, and are easy to implement (Cohen et al., 1991; Bedimo et al., in review). While these types of campaigns should not replace individual and community-level risk reduction interventions, they can be strong complements to the prevention efforts made by those more intensive programs (Bedimo et al., in review). Both individual-level and population-based interventions should be used to prevent the further spread of HIV (Kelly, 1999).

Similarly, prevention social marketing has been effective in reducing risk behavior in both industrialized countries, such as Switzerland (Dubois-Arber et al., 1997), and developing countries, such as Thailand (Nelson et al., 1996). In the United States, the only AIDS-related nationwide mass media campaign to date was "America Responds to AIDS" (ARTA). Conducted from October 1987 to July 1990, ARTA was a five-phased multimedia (e.g., multilingual mailings, public service announcements on television and radio stations, and posters) campaign designed to increase public awareness of and knowledge about HIV/AIDS. A smaller-scale social marketing effort, the Prevention Marketing Initiative, was implemented by the CDC in 1994 and was directed at adolescents in five cities. This initiative was successful in obtaining positive behavioral risk-reduction outcomes among adolescents, such as increases in carrying condoms and reductions in the number of unprotected sexual acts (U.S. Conference of Mayors, 1994; Kennedy et al., 2000). Broader implementation of such programs in the United States could potentially reach those risk populations who have limited or sporadic access to HIV prevention messages. Further, educational components of such campaigns can help to reduce the stigma and negative attitudes associated with HIV/AIDS, substance abuse, and sexuality.

There also is striking evidence in support of policy interventions that increase individuals' access to prevention services and tools. For example, needle-exchange programs have been widely demonstrated to be effective in reducing substance use-related risk behaviors (such as needle sharing) without increasing overall prevalence of substance use in either adults or youth (e.g., IOM, 1995; Valleroy et al., 1995). Unfortunately, societal interventions are underutilized in the United States due to social attitudes and policy barriers opposing their implementation. These barriers are addressed in greater detail in Chapter 7.

REFERENCES USED IN THE COMPLILATION OF THE TABLE OF BIOMEDICAL AND BEHAVIORAL INTERVENTIONS

AIDS Community Demonstration Projects. 1999. Community-level HIV intervention in 5 cities: Final outcome data from the CDC AIDS Community Demonstration Projects. *American Journal of Public Health* 89(3):336–345.

Andreasen AR. 1995. *Marketing Social Change*. San Francisco: Jossey-Bass.

Bedimo AL, Pinkerton SD, Cohen DA, Gray B, Farley TA. In review. Cost-savings of a condom social marketing program. *American Journal of Public Health*.

Bhave G, Lindan CP, Hudes ES, Desai S, Wagle U, Tripathi SP, Mandel JS. 1995. Impact of an intervention on HIV, sexually transmitted diseases, and condom use among sex workers in Bombay, India. *AIDS* 9 (Suppl 1):S21–S30.

Booth RE and Watters JK. 1994. How effective are risk-reduction interventions targeting injecting drug users? *AIDS* 8(11):1515–1524.

Boyer CB, Barrett DC, Peterman TA, Bolan G. 1997. Sexually transmitted disease (STD) and HIV risk in heterosexual adults attending a public STD clinic: Evaluation of a randomized controlled behavioral risk-reduction intervention trial. *AIDS* 11(3):359–367.

Centers for Disease Control and Prevention (CDC). 1996. Update: Provisional Public Health Service recommendations for chemoprophylaxis after occupational exposure to HIV. *Morbidity and Mortality Weekly Report* 45(22):468–480.

Centers for Disease Control and Prevention (CDC). 1998. The CDC-sponsored External Consultants Meeting on Antiretroviral Therapy for Potential Nonoccupational Exposures to HIV; Jul 24–25, 1997; Atlanta (Web Page). Located at: www.cdc.gov/nchstp/hiv_aids/media/pepfact3.htm.

Centers for Disease Control and Prevention (CDC), Prevention Research Synthesis Project. 1999. Compendium of HIV prevention interventions with evidence of effectiveness. (Web Page). Located at: www.cdc.gov/hiv/projects/rep/compend.htm.

Cheever LW, Keruly JC, Moore RD. 1998. A new program to improve adherence with HIV treatment (Abstract I-217). Interscience Conference on Antimicrobial Agents and Chemotherapy; Sep 24–27, 1998.

Cohen D, Dent C, MacKinnon D. 1991. Condom skills education and sexually transmitted disease reinfection. *Journal of Sex Research* 28(1):139–144.

Cohen MS. 1995. HIV and sexually transmitted diseases. The physician's role in prevention. *Postgraduate Medicine* 98(3):52–58, 63–64.

Connor EM, Sperling RS, Gelber R, Kiselev P, Scott G, O'Sullivan MJ, VanDyke R, Bey M, Shearer W, Jacobson RL, Jimenez E, O'Neill E, Bazin B, Delfraissy JF, Culnane M, Coombs R, Elkins M, Moye J, Stratton P, Balsley J. 1994. Reduction of maternal–infant transmission of human immunodeficiency virus type 1 with zidovudine treatment. Pediatric AIDS Clinical Trials Group Protocol 076 Study Group. *New England Journal of Medicine* 331(18):1173–1180.

DiClemente RJ, Wingood GM. 1995. A randomized controlled trial of an HIV sexual risk-reduction intervention for young African-American women. *Journal of the American Medical Association* 274(16):1271–1276.

Drake RE, Osher FC. 1997. Treating substance abuse in patients with severe mental illness. In Henggeler SW and Santos AB (Eds.), *Innovative Approaches for Difficult-to-Treat Populations*. Washington, DC: American Psychiatric Press.

Dubois-Arber F, Jeannin A, Konings E, Paccaud F. 1997. Increased condom use without other major changes in sexual behavior among the general population in Switzerland. *American Journal of Public Health* 87(4):558–566.

Exner TM, Gardos PS, Seal DW, Ehrhardt AA. 1999. HIV sexual risk reduction interventions with heterosexual men: The forgotten group. *AIDS and Behavior* 3(4):347–358.

Exner TM, Seal DW, Ehrhardt AA. 1997. A review of HIV interventions for at-risk women. *AIDS and Behavior* 1(2):93–124.

Folkman S, Chesney MA, Pollack L, Phillips C. 1992. Stress, coping, and high-risk sexual behavior. *Health Psychology* 11(4):218–222.

Ford K and Norris AE. 1993. Knowledge of AIDS transmission, risk behavior, and perceptions of risk among urban, low-income, African-American and Hispanic youth. *American Journal of Preventive Medicine* 9(5):297–306.

Ford K, Wirawan DN, Fajans P, Meliawan P, MacDonald K, Thorpe L. 1996. Behavioral interventions for reduction of sexually transmitted disease/HIV transmission among female commercial sex workers and clients in Bali, Indonesia. *AIDS* 10(2):213–222.

Holtgrave DR, Pinkerton SD, Jones TS, Lurie P, Vlahov D. 1998. Cost and cost-effectiveness of increasing access to sterile syringes and needles as an HIV prevention intervention in the United States. *Journal of Acquired Immune Deficiency Syndromes and Human Retrovirology* 18(Suppl 1):S133–S138.

Iguchi MY. 1998. Drug abuse treatment as HIV prevention: Changes in social drug use patterns might also reduce risk. *Journal of Addictive Diseases* 17(4):9–18.

Institute of Medicine. 1995. *HIV and the Blood Supply: An Analysis of Crisis Decisionmaking.* Leviton L, Sox HC, and Stoto MA (Eds.). Washington, DC: National Academy Press.

Institute of Medicine. 1999. *Reducing the Odds: Preventing Perinatal Transmission of HIV in the United States.* Stoto MA, Almario DA, and McCormick MC (Eds.). Washington, DC: National Academy Press.

Jemmott JB 3rd, Jemmott LS, Fong GT. 1992. Reductions in HIV risk-associated sexual behaviors among black male adolescents: Effects of an AIDS prevention intervention. *American Journal of Public Health* 82(3):372–377.

Jemmott JB 3rd, Jemmott LS, Fong GT. 1998. Abstinence and safer sex HIV risk-reduction interventions for African American adolescents: a randomized controlled trial. *Journal of the American Medical Association* 279(19):1529–1536.

Kamb ML, Fishbein M, Douglas JM Jr, Rhodes F, Rogers J, Bolan G, Zenilman J, Hoxworth T, Malotte CK, Iatesta M, Kent C, Lentz A, Graziano S, Byers RH, Peterman TA. 1998. Efficacy of risk-reduction counseling to prevent human immunodeficiency virus and sexually transmitted diseases: A randomized controlled trial. Project RESPECT Study Group. *Journal of the American Medical Association* 280(13):1161–1167.

Kegeles SM, Hays RB, Coates TJ. 1996. The Mpowerment Project: A community-level HIV prevention intervention for young gay men. *American Journal of Public Health* 86(8 Pt 1):1129–1136.

Kelly JA. 1999. Community-level interventions are needed to prevent new HIV infections. *American Journal of Public Health* 89(3):299–301.

Kelly JA, St. Lawrence JS, Stevenson LY, Hauth AC, Kalichman SC, Diaz YE, Brasfield TL, Koob JJ, Morgan MG. 1992. Community AIDS/HIV risk reduction: The effects of endorsements by popular people in three cities. *American Journal of Public Health* 82(11):1483–1489.

Kennedy MG, Mizuno Y, Hoffman R, Baume C, Strand J. 2000. The effect of tailoring a model HIV prevention program for local adolescent target audiences. *AIDS Education and Prevention* 12(3):225–238.

Magura S, Kang SY, Shapiro JL. 1994. Outcomes of intensive AIDS education for male adolescent drug users in jail. *Journal of Adolescent Health* 15(6):457–463.

Main DS, Iverson DC, McGloin J, Banspach SW, Collins JL, Rugg DL, Kolbe LJ. 1994. Preventing HIV infection among adolescents: evaluation of a school-based education program. *Preventive Medicine* 23(4):409–417.

Marks G, Bingman C, Duval S. 1998. Negative affect and unsafe sex in HIV-positive men. *AIDS and Behavior* 2(2):89–99.

Moss AR, Vranizan K, Gorter R, Bacchetti P, Watters J, Osmond D. 1994. HIV seroconversion in intravenous drug users in San Francisco, 1985–1990. *AIDS* 8(2):223–231.

Murphy DA, Wilson C, Durako S, Muenz L, Belzer M. 1999. Antiretroviral medication adherence among the REACH HIV-infected adolescent cohort (Abstract 152). National HIV Prevention Conference; August 29–September 1, 1999; Atlanta.

The National Institute of Mental Health (NIMH) Multisite HIV Prevention Trial Group. 1998. The NIMH Multisite HIV Prevention Trial: Reducing HIV sexual risk behavior. *Science* 280(5371):1889–1894.

National Institutes of Health. 1997. Interventions to prevent HIV risk behaviors. *NIH Consensus Statement* 15(2):1–41.

Nelson KE, Celentano DD, Eiumtrakol S, Hoover DR, Beyrer C, Suprasert S, Kuntolbutra S, Khamboonruang C. 1996. Changes in sexual behavior and a decline in HIV infection among young men in Thailand. *New England Journal of Medicine* 335(5):297–303.

Ngugi EN, Plummer FA, Simonsen JN, Cameron DW, Bosire M, Waiyaki P, Ronald AR, Ndinya-Achola JO. 1988. Prevention of transmission of human immunodeficiency virus in Africa: effectiveness of condom promotion and health education among prostitutes. *Lancet* 2(8616):887–890.

Pinkerton SD and Holtgrave DR. 1998. The cost-effectiveness of HIV prevention from a managed care perspective. *Journal of Public Health Management and Practice* 4(1):59–66.

Quinn TC, Wawer MJ, Sewankambo N, Serwadda D, Li C, Wabwire-Mangen F, Meehan MO, Lutalo T, Gray RH. 2000. Viral load and heterosexual transmission of human immunodeficiency virus type 1. Rakai Project Study Group. *New England Journal of Medicine* 342(13):921–929.

Regier DA, Narrow WE, Rae DS, Manderscheid RW, Locke BZ, Goodwin FK. 1993. The de facto US mental and addictive disorders service system. Epidemiologic catchment area prospective 1-year prevalence rates of disorders and services. *Archives of General Psychiatry* 50(2):85–94.

Rotheram-Borus MJ, Gillis JR, Reid HM, Fernandez MI, Gwadz M. 1997. HIV testing, behaviors, and knowledge among adolescents at high risk. *Journal of Adolescent Health* 20(3):216–225.

Schulz RM, Mullenix TA, Googe HL, Grant D, Duong PT, Ortiz E. 1998. Depression scores and antiretroviral therapy adherence in HIV disease (Abstract I-215). Interscience Conference on Antimicrobial Agents and Chemotherapy; Sep 24–27, 1998; San Diego.

Shoptaw S, Reback CJ, Frosch DL, Rawson RA. 1998. Stimulant abuse treatment as HIV prevention. *Journal of Addictive Diseases* 17(4):19–32.

Sikkema KJ, Kelly JA, Winett RA, Solomon LJ, Cargill VA, Roffman RA, McAuliffe TL, Heckman TG, Anderson EA, Wagstaff DA, Norman AD, Perry MJ, Crumble DA, Mercer MB. 2000. Outcomes of a randomized community-level HIV prevention intervention for women living in 18 low-income housing developments. *American Journal of Public Health* 90(1):57–63.

St. Lawrence JS, Brasfield TL, Jefferson KW, Alleyne E, O'Bannon RE 3rd, Shirley A. 1995. Cognitive-behavioral intervention to reduce African American adolescents' risk for HIV infection. *Journal of Consulting and Clinical Psychology* 63(2):221–237.

Stanton BF, Li X, Ricardo I, Galbraith J, Feigelman S, Kaljee L. 1996. A randomized, controlled effectiveness trial of an AIDS prevention program for low-income African-American youths. *Archives of Pediatric and Adolescent Medicine* 150(4):363–372.

U.S. Conference of Mayors. 1994. CDC's Prevention Marketing Initiative: A Multi-level Approach to HIV Prevention. *HIV Capsule Report*, Issue 2. Washington, DC: U.S. Conference of Mayors.

Valdiserri RO, Lyter DW, Leviton LC, Callahan CM, Kingsley LA, Rinaldo CR. 1989. AIDS prevention in homosexual and bisexual men: Results of a randomized trial evaluating two risk reduction interventions. *AIDS* 3(1):21–26.

Valleroy LA, Weinstein B, Jones TS, Groseclose SL, Rolfs RT, Kassler WJ. 1995. Impact of increased legal access to needles and syringes on community pharmacies' needle and syringe sales—Connecticut, 1992. *Journal of Acquired Immune Deficiency Syndromes and Human Retrovirology* 10(1):73–81.

C

Federal Spending on HIV/AIDS

OVERVIEW OF FEDERAL HIV/AIDS SPENDING

Since HIV/AIDS was first recognized in the United States in 1981, annual federal spending has grown from an appropriation of several hundred thousand dollars to more than $9.7 billion in fiscal year (FY) 1999. Of this 1999 amount, $6.9 billion (71 percent) was spent on care and assistance for people with HIV/AIDS, $1.9 billion (19 percent) on research, $775.3 million (8 percent) on prevention, and $142 million (2 percent) on international efforts (Figure C.1)[1] (Foster et al., 1999).

Spending for prevention efforts, in terms of both absolute spending and percentage increases, has lagged far behind investments in HIV/ AIDS-related care and assistance programs and research. From FY95 through FY99, real spending for care and assistance programs increased by 42 percent, while spending for research increased by 21 percent. In contrast, real spending on prevention remained relatively flat, with only a 9 percent increase during this same period (Figure C.2) (Foster et al., 1999).

Federal spending on HIV/AIDS is enormously complex and divided

---

[1]For more detailed information on FY99 federal HIV/AIDS spending and trends, see Foster et al. (1999), *Federal HIV/AIDS Spending: A Budget Chartbook*. Report prepared for the Kaiser Family Foundation.

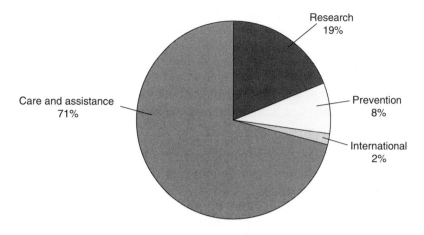

Total expenditure: $9.7 billion

FIGURE C.1 Fiscal Year 1999 federal HIV/AIDS spending.

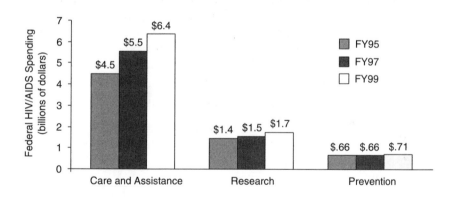

FIGURE C.2 Fiscal Year 1995–1999 domestic federal HIV/AIDS spending (in billions of 1996 dollars). SOURCE: Nominal HIV/AIDS spending data from Foster et al. (1999). Price deflators provided by the Bureau of Labor Statistics.

among many different departments and agencies within the federal government. The Department of Health and Human Services (DHHS) and its respective agencies account for approximately 75 percent of spending on prevention, research, and treatment. Other departments and agencies outside of DHHS with a role in HIV/AIDS prevention, research, and treatment include: the Social Security Administration ($1.1 billion), the Department of Veterans Affairs ($403 million), the Department of Housing and Urban Development ($225 million), the U.S. Agency for International Development ($135 million), the Department of Defense ($107 million), the Department of Justice ($7 million), the Peace Corps ($5 million), the Department of Labor ($2 million), and the U.S. Information Agency ($0.7 million) (Foster et al., 1999).

OVERVIEW OF DEPARTMENT OF HEALTH AND HUMAN SERVICES SPENDING ON HIV/AIDS

This section describes DHHS's operating divisions that are involved in primary and secondary HIV prevention and research. It also briefly discusses DHHS agencies whose primary function is care and assistance (e.g., the Health Care Financing Administration and the Health Resources Services Administration), as these agencies have a role in expanding prevention efforts to the clinical setting (see Chapter 4).

The spending figures reported in this section were obtained from a variety of sources, but primarily came from budgets and other documents submitted by the federal agencies. The Committee did not independently verify these figures, nor did we attempt to reconcile budgets across agencies using a common definition of prevention. As a result, there is some inconsistency across agencies with respect to the types of activities that are categorized under the heading of prevention.

Centers for Disease Control and Prevention

The Centers for Disease Control and Prevention (CDC) directs and oversees the nation's largest and most comprehensive group of federally funded HIV prevention programs. Responsibility for these programs is divided among eight centers, institutes, and offices. HIV prevention efforts are primarily concentrated in two divisions of the National Center for HIV, STD, and TB Prevention: the Division of HIV/AIDS Prevention–Intervention Research and Support and the Division of HIV/AIDS Prevention–Surveillance and Epidemiology.

In FY99, the CDC spent $678 million on HIV-related activities (CDC, 1999b). The CDC's FY99 HIV/AIDS funding can be divided into the following six major categories (CDC, 1999c):

• *Intervention/Program Implementation*: In FY99, the CDC distributed $412 million of its HIV budget externally through cooperative agreements, grants, and contracts, to states and localities for prevention services. Approximately two-thirds of this amount ($258 million) was distributed through external cooperative agreements with 65 state and select local health departments to support prevention activities such as health education and risk reduction programs and counseling and testing services (CDC, 1999c). Priorities for use of these funds are set by Community Planning Groups, comprised of representatives from groups at risk for HIV infection and providers of HIV prevention services. In addition, the CDC supports HIV prevention programs through grants and competitive funding processes for 22 national and regional minority organizations; 10 national business, labor, and faith partnerships; and 94 community-based organizations (CDC, 1999a).

• *Surveillance*: The CDC supports a variety of epidemiological and behavioral surveillance activities to monitor HIV/AIDS-related trends, such as HIV and AIDS cases, AIDS deaths, risk behaviors, HIV-related knowledge, and HIV testing behaviors (CDC, 1999a). Approximately $72.3 million (11 percent) of total FY99 program funding was used for surveillance activities (CDC, 1999c).

• *Research:* The CDC conducts biomedical and behavioral prevention research for a number of areas including preventing HIV transmission, mechanisms of HIV infection and disease progression, HIV and STD treatment, and microbicides and vaccines (CDC, 1999a). FY99 funding for research activities was $88.1 million (14 percent of total funding) (CDC, 1999c).

• *Technical Assistance:* In FY99, approximately $51.7 million (8 percent of total funding) was used for technical assistance, training, capacity building, and information dissemination (CDC, 1999c).

• *Program Evaluation*: In FY99, approximately $11.9 million (2 percent of total funding) was used for program evaluation (CDC, 1999c).

• *Policy:* In FY99, approximately $1.6 million (<.01 percent of total funding) was used for policy development (CDC, 1999c).

National Institutes of Health

The National Institutes of Health (NIH) is the primary research arm of DHHS. The NIH is comprised of 25 separate institutes and centers, all of which are involved in HIV/AIDS-related research activities. The institutes and centers whose programs are most heavily concerned with HIV/AIDS include: the National Cancer Institute, the National Institute for Drug Abuse, the National Institute of Mental Health, the National Center for Research Resources, the National Heart, Lung and Blood Institute, the National Institute of Child Health and Human Development, and the National Institute of Allergy and Infectious Diseases (OAR, 1999).

In 1988, NIH established the Office of AIDS Research (OAR) to coordinate its AIDS research and to serve as a focal point for AIDS policy and budget development. The OAR has established and supports the efforts of six trans-NIH Coordinating Committees in each of the following areas: Natural History and Epidemiology, Etiology and Pathogenesis, Therapeutics, Vaccines, Behavioral and Social Sciences, and Information Dissemination. Prevention studies are found in each of these primary research areas. The NIH and OAR also provide support in training, infrastructure, and capacity building (OAR, 1999).

NIH's FY99 budget for AIDS-related research was approximately $1.8 billion. The NIH reports that approximately one-third of its AIDS-related research budget supports both nonvaccine-related and vaccine-related prevention research (OAR, 2000a).

Nonvaccine Prevention Research

In FY99, $359 million (20 percent of total funding) supported studies of and interventions for primary prevention, which examined the factors, determinants, and processes of HIV risk and transmission. Approximately $181 million (6 percent of total funding) supported studies of and interventions for secondary prevention of HIV/AIDS, which examined biological and behavioral factors that influence disease progression and the negative psychosocial consequences of HIV/AIDS (OAR, 2000a).

In FY97, NIH began an HIV Prevention Science Initiative to promote comprehensive, crossdisciplinary HIV prevention science. Each year, OAR, with assistance from the Prevention Science Working Group, identifies prevention science priorities and develops a research agenda to address opportunities and gaps in nonvaccine HIV prevention science. Major priority areas of the Initiative from FY97 through FY99 have included the following (OAR, 2000b):

• **FY97** Impact of new therapies on HIV prevention; primary/acute infection; prevention of perinatal transmission; comprehensive HIV prevention strategies for injection drug users; and biobehavioral issues in the development and utilization of HIV prevention methods under female control.

• **FY98** *Primary priority:* Impact of early identification, counseling, and other behavioral interventions, HIV treatment on risk behaviors, the utilization of HIV prevention services, and the transmission of HIV. *Secondary priorities:* Comprehensive HIV prevention strategies for substance users; strategies for preventing vertical transmission of HIV; and prevention methods for women.

• **FY99** *Primary priority:* HIV prevention among racial and ethnic minorities. *Secondary priorities:* Relationship between biological and behavioral outcomes; sustainability of HIV prevention efforts; international HIV prevention research; legal, ethical, and policy issues in HIV prevention; and primary prevention for men who have sex with women.

Vaccine Research

Approximately 10 percent ($182 million) of NIH's AIDS-related budget supports basic, preclinical, and clinical research on candidate vaccine products (OAR, 2000a). The NIH also supports the Innovative Vaccine Grants Program, which provides one or two years of funding to investigators to explore new concepts in basic research related to AIDS vaccines. In addition, a cross-institute NIH Vaccine Research Center has been initiated, and which will be funded by intramural programs of the National Institute of Allergy and Infectious Diseases and the National Cancer Institute (NIH, 1999).

Substance Abuse and Mental Health Administration

The Substance Abuse and Mental Health Administration (SAMHSA) is the agency within DHHS with primary responsibility for supporting substance abuse treatment and prevention and mental health services. SAMHSA is comprised of three centers: the Center for Mental Health Services (CMHS), the Center for Substance Abuse Prevention (CSAP), and the Center for Substance Abuse Treatment (CSAT). The Agency's current HIV/AIDS-related activities include:

- *SAPT Block Grant*: The Substance Abuse Prevention and Treatment (SAPT) block grant is the largest program administered by SAMHSA, with approximately $1.6 billion in funding in FY99. Ninety-five percent of the SAPT block grant funds are distributed to states and territories, based on a formula established by Congress, to support substance abuse treatment and prevention services (SAMHSA, 2000b). While Congress provides general direction on how funds can be used, states have broad discretion in allocating these funds. Currently, however, little information exists about how the funds are used by states or about the effectiveness of programs that are funded. Efforts are under way to determine the outcomes of states' programs (GAO, 2000).
- *SAPT Block Grant-Funded Early Intervention Services (HIV Set-Aside)*: As part of the ADAMHA Reorganization Act of 1992 (P.L. 102-321), Congress enacted a provision that requires states with an AIDS case rate of 10 or more per 100,000 population to use a portion (2–5 percent) of their SAPT block grant funding for early HIV-intervention services (SAMHSA, 2000b). These prevention activities may include: HIV education and risk reduction, counseling and testing, diagnostic services and assessment,

and medical consultation (SAMHSA, 1999). In FY99, 26 states set aside $54 million under this provision for HIV-related prevention efforts (SAMHSA, 2000a). As with the SAPT block grant, however, little information exists about how these funds are used or the effectiveness of programs sponsored by states.

• *Knowledge Development and Application (KDA) Programs:* KDA programs are designed to help translate promising evidence-based prevention and treatment interventions from the controlled research environment into community settings. Examples of HIV-related KDA programs and studies include: the HIV Cost Study, the HIV/AIDS High Risk Behavior Prevention/Intervention Model for Youth Adult/Adolescent and Women Program, and the Center for Substance Abuse Prevention's HIV Prevention Initiative for Youth and Women of Color (SAMHSA, 2000b).[2]

• *Targeted Capacity Expansion and HIV Outreach Grants:* SAMHSA's Targeted Capacity Expansion (TCE) program provides grants to state and local governments to address emerging and urgent substance abuse treatment and prevention needs of racial and ethnic minorities and other vulnerable populations. In addition, as part of the FY99 Congressional Black Caucus initiative, CSAT began implementing community-based substance abuse and HIV/AIDS outreach program grants, targeting minority communities with high rates of substance abuse and HIV/AIDS. Services funded under this program include outreach, HIV counseling and testing, health education and risk reduction information, access and referrals to testing for sexually transmitted diseases and tuberculosis, substance abuse treatment, primary care, and mental health and medical services. In FY99, CSAT administered $39 million in TCE and outreach grants to enhance and expand substance abuse treatment and services related to HIV/AIDS (SAMHSA, 2000c).

Health Resources and Services Administration

The Health Resources and Services Administration (HRSA) provides health care services to underserved, uninsured, and underinsured communities and individuals. The Agency has lead responsibility for administering the Ryan White CARE Act, which is the largest financial allocation specifically for HIV-related health care and support services. Programs under the CARE Act are managed by HRSA's Bureau of HIV/AIDS.

---

[2]No funding figures were available for HIV-specific related KDA programs.

The Ryan White CARE Act

The Ryan White Comprehensive AIDS Resources Emergency (CARE) Act of 1990 (P.L.101-381) was passed in response to the growing AIDS epidemic. The Act was reauthorized in 1996 (P.L. 104-146) and is currently undergoing a subsequent reauthorization. The CARE Act is specifically designed to serve HIV-infected individuals who have fallen through the existing public safety net. The Act is the official "payer of last resort" and can be used only when no other funding source is available to pay for services (HRSA, 2000).

Annual funding for the CARE Act has increased substantially since its inception, from approximately $220 million in FY91 to approximately $1.4 billion in FY99. In FY99, the CARE Act accounted for 19 percent of total federal HIV/AIDS spending. In FY98, the majority of CARE Act funds were used for health care services (30 percent) and medications (34 percent). Twelve percent was used for support services (e.g., transportation, food, and emergency housing assistance), 8 percent for case management, 8 percent for planning and evaluation, and the remainder for other programs (HRSA, 2000).

The CARE Act provides assistance under four program "titles" and through Part F. Titles I–III account for 95 percent of the Act's FY99 appropriations (HRSA, 2000).

- *Title I: Grants to Eligible Metropolitan Areas.* Title I provides emergency relief grants to Eligible Metropolitan Areas (EMAs) that have been disproportionately affected by the HIV epidemic.[3] An HIV Health Services Planning Council sets priorities for the allocation of funds within the EMA based on service gaps within their region. In FY99, $505.2 million was provided under Title I grants to 51 EMAs (HRSA, 2000).
- *Title II: Grants to States and Territories.* Title II provides formula grants to all 50 states, the District of Columbia, Puerto Rico, Guam, and the U.S. Virgin Islands for health care and support services for people living with HIV disease. Title II also provides access to pharmaceuticals through the AIDS Drug Assistance Program (ADAP). In recent years, an increasing portion of Title II grants has been "earmarked" by Congress to fund medications through ADAP, increasing from $167 million in FY97 to $461 million in FY99. In FY99, $738 million was provided under Title II, with $277 million for grants to states and territories and $461 million for ADAPs (HRSA, 2000).

---

[3]To be eligible, an area must have more than 2,000 cumulative AIDS cases reported during the past 5 years, and have a population of at least 500,000.

- *Title III: Early Intervention Grants.* Title III provides grants to expand the service capacity of organizations providing primary care services to indigent HIV-positive individuals. Title III programs are funded to provide early intervention services that include: risk reduction counseling; partner involvement in risk reduction; education to prevent transmission; antibody testing; medical evaluation; and clinical care; antiretroviral therapies; protection against opportunistic infections; case management; and interventions to address "co-epidemics," including tuberculosis and substance abuse. In FY99, $94.3 million was provided in early intervention grants under Title III (HRSA, 2000).

- *Title IV: Women, Infants, Children, and Youth.* Title IV provides comprehensive, community-based services to children, youth, and women, who are either at-risk for or living with HIV. Title IV program services include primary and specialty medical care, psychosocial services, logistical support, outreach, and prevention. Title IV systems of care provide access to and linkage with clinical research and trials. In FY99, $46 million was provided to support 58 grants and three initiatives addressing problems in children, adolescents, and women living with HIV (HRSA, 2000).

- *Other Programs (Part F):*

  (1)   fourteen AIDS Education Training Centers that offer HIV/AIDS training and education to clinicians across the country (FY99 funding of $20 million);

  (2)   Special Projects of National Significance, which implement and evaluate models that can be replicated throughout the country for reaching underserved populations and delivering HIV care (FY99 funding of $25 million); and

  (3)   Dental Reimbursement Program, which provides funds to offset the cost of uncompensated HIV care in teaching institutions, to improve access to oral health care, and to help train dental students and residents in caring for persons with HIV (FY99 funding of $7.8 million) (HRSA, 2000).

Food and Drug Administration

The Food and Drug Administration (FDA) has several centers and offices that are involved in HIV prevention from a regulatory perspective. The FDA is responsible for ensuring the safety and efficacy of blood and blood products, and is the principal regulatory authority regarding blood and blood products, including blood banking practices, the handling of source plasma, and the manufacture of blood products from plasma. The FDA is also responsible for the regulation and licensing of vaccines to treat or prevent HIV infection. In addition, FDA regulates topical microbicides and drugs to prevent perinatal transmission of HIV. The

FDA plays a primary role in the regulation and development of barrier products, such as condoms and surgical and examination gloves (FDA, 2000). In FY99, FDA spent an estimated $76.7 million on HIV/AIDS related efforts, with $21.8 million devoted to prevention and $54.9 million to research (Foster et al., 1999).

Health Care Financing Administration

The Health Care Financing Administration (HCFA) administers the Medicaid and Medicare programs, both of which are major sources of financing for HIV/AIDS-related medical care and assistance.

Medicaid

Medicaid is a jointly funded, federal–state health insurance program for certain low-income and medically needy individuals. Medicaid is the single largest payer of direct medical services for people living with AIDS, serving over 50 percent of all persons living with AIDS and up to 90 percent of all children with AIDS (Westmoreland, 1999). Individuals with HIV are generally not eligible for Medicaid; however, Maine was granted a demonstration waiver by HCFA in February 2000 to extend Medicaid benefits to nondisabled persons living with HIV disease (Kaiser Family Foundation, 2000). States are required to provide the full range of Medicaid services covered in the state plan to eligible persons with HIV disease, but have the option of providing services such as targeted case management, preventive services, and hospice care. In FY99, combined federal and state Medicaid expenditures were $3.9 billion. Federal Medicaid expenditures, which totaled $2.1 billion, accounted for 22 percent of total federal spending on HIV/AIDS in FY99 (Foster et al., 1999).

Medicare

Medicare is the nation's largest health insurance program; it covers 39 million persons who are age 65 and over or who have certain disabilities. In FY99, Medicare provided $1.5 billion in care and assistance to individuals with HIV/AIDS (Foster et al., 1999).

Other DHHS Agencies with HIV/AIDS Spending:

- *Indian Health Service*: The Agency spent an estimated $3.6 million on HIV/AIDS prevention programs for American Indians and Alaskan Natives in FY99[4] (Foster et al., 1999).

---

[4]No separate estimates for Care and Assistance programs were available.

• *Agency for Health Care Quality and Research*: The Agency spent an estimated $1.5 million on research programs for HIV/AIDS (Foster et al., 1999).

REFERENCES

Centers for Disease Control and Prevention (CDC). 1999a. CDC's HIV/AIDS Prevention Activities. Atlanta: CDC.

Centers for Disease Control and Prevention (CDC). 1999b. Chart: HIV Prevention Funding FY 94–99. Atlanta: CDC.

Centers for Disease Control and Prevention (CDC). 1999c. Provisional Project List by Mission Category for FY 99 CDC HIV/AIDS Budget. Atlanta: CDC.

Food and Drug Administration. 2000. Testimony of Birnkrant D, Egan W, Klein R, and Tabor E, to the Institute of Medicine's Committee on HIV Prevention Strategies, March 1, 2000, Washington, DC.

Foster S, Gregory A, Niederhausen P, Rapallo D, Westmoreland T. 1999. *Federal HIV/AIDS Spending: A Budget Chartbook*. Report Prepared for the Kaiser Family Foundation. Washington, DC: Georgetown University Law Center.

Health Resources and Services Administration (HRSA), HIV/AIDS Bureau. 2000. *The AIDS Epidemic and the Ryan White CARE Act: Past Progress, Future Challenges*. Washington, DC: HRSA.

Kaiser Family Foundation. 2000. *Project Description: Medicaid Eligibility Expansion for People with HIV Prior to Disability*. Menlo Park, CA: Kaiser Family Foundation.

National Institutes of Health (NIH). 1999. AIDS Research on HIV Prevention: FY 1999 Estimated. Bethesda, MD: NIH.

Office of AIDS Research (OAR), National Institutes of Health. 1999. *National Institutes of Health Fiscal Year 2001 Plan for HIV-Related Research*. Bethesda, MD: NIH.

Office of AIDS Research (OAR), National Institutes of Health. 2000a. NIH AIDS Research on HIV Prevention: FY99 Estimated. Document prepared for the Committee on HIV Prevention Strategies. (Received in e-mail communication from Judith Auerbach, March 3, 2000.)

Office of AIDS Research (OAR), National Institutes of Health. 2000b. OAR Prevention Science Initiative Awards by Priority Areas (FY97–FY99). Document prepared for the Committee on HIV Prevention Strategies. (Received in e-mail communication from Judith Auerbach, March 3, 2000.)

Substance Abuse and Mental Health Services Administration (SAMHSA). 1999. SAMHSA/CSAT Fact Sheet on the HIV Set-Aside of the Substance Abuse Prevention and Treatment Block Grant. Washington, DC: SAMHSA.

Substance Abuse and Mental Health Services Administration (SAMHSA). 2000a. "HIV Designated States" Fiscal Year Obligations, Substance Abuse Prevention and Treatment Block Grant. Washington, DC: SAMHSA.

Substance Abuse and Mental Health Services Administration (SAMHSA). 2000b. *HIV Strategic Plan*. Washington, DC: SAMHSA.

Substance Abuse and Mental Health Services Administration (SAMHSA). 2000c. Targeted Capacity Expansion Program for Substance Abuse Treatment and HIV/AIDS Services. Washington, DC: SAMHSA.

United States General Accounting Office (GAO) 2000. *Drug Abuse Treatment: Efforts Under Way to Determine Effectiveness of State Programs* (GAO/HEHS-00-50). Washington, DC: GAO.

Westmoreland T. 1999. *Medicaid and HIV/AIDS Policy: A Basic Primer*. Report Prepared for the Kaiser Family Foundation. Washington, DC: Federal Legislation Clinic, Georgetown University Law Center.

D
Description and Mathematical Statement of the HIV Prevention Resource Allocation Model

Thus appendix presents a brief description and mathematical statement of the model the Committee used to produce the examples discussed in Chapter 3. The Committee structured our analysis around four steps, which are briefly described below: estimating aggregate HIV incidence, estimating the efficacy and reach of HIV prevention programs, estimating the costs of HIV prevention, and allocating the HIV prevention budget to prevent as many new infections as possible.

ESTIMATING AGGREGATE HIV INCIDENCE

HIV incidence data broken down by location and HIV risk group are sorely lacking. The only description the Committee found of a systematic attempt to provide such estimates was a paper in the *American Journal of Public Health* (Holmberg, 1996). Our analysis uses estimates of HIV incidence broken down by injection drug users, men who have sex with men, and high-risk heterosexuals for 96 Standard Metropolitan Statistical Areas in the United States, aggregated to the state level. As discussed in Chapter 2 in this report, however, the systematic estimation of HIV incidence remains a crucial data need to effectively plan and evaluate HIV prevention programs.

ESTIMATING THE EFFICACY AND REACH
OF HIV PREVENTION PROGRAMS

The Committee reviewed peer-reviewed publications reporting evaluations of HIV prevention programs. It has proven challenging to interpret such studies in terms of the relative reduction in the rate of new HIV infections implied by the programs examined. Yet, it is precisely this information about new infections that is required to sensibly consider the overall impact of alternative plans for distributing HIV prevention dollars.

To develop data for this analysis, we reviewed in detail a subset of HIV prevention studies with an eye toward estimating the relative reduction in exposure to HIV risk as a result of prevention interventions aimed at men who have sex with men, injection drug users, and women at high risk for heterosexual transmission (see references at the end of this appendix for a listing of the studies reviewed). These three risk groups were selected to coincide with the risk group classification employed by Holmberg in estimating HIV incidence (Holmberg, 1996). Prevention efficacy, defined as the percentage reduction in new HIV infections, was estimated under the assumption that HIV incidence is proportional to the product of HIV prevalence and risky exposure rates (or "contact rates," as defined in the mathematical epidemiology literature; see Anderson and May, 1991, and Kahn, 1996, for an example). There is little question that more work along these lines is needed in order to better understand the value of HIV prevention interventions.

The Committee's review of these studies also revealed that there were the high rates of subject attrition from the interventions evaluated. This observation led us to question the ability of many prevention programs to effectively reach and retain program participants over time. An intervention might be effective for program participants, but unable to reach more than, say, 10 percent of the total population. While many discussions of HIV prevention assume, in fact, that all persons at risk can be contacted, the Committee felt it was important to build into the analysis the recognition that not all of those at risk can be reached by interventions. Because no data exist on program reach, the Committee made some assumptions in the analysis to account for this fact. We assumed: 50 percent in the base case; 75 percent in the optimistic case; and 25 percent in the pessimistic case.

THE COSTS OF HIV PREVENTION PROGRAMS

The Committee notes that very few evaluations of HIV prevention programs report the costs of providing such services, though there are some exceptions (see Holtgrave, 1998). For each of the HIV prevention studies reviewed, a research assistant working with the Committee produced an estimate of the average cost per client enrolled, using resource-based costing (see Gorsky, 1996, for a description of the approach). Typical resources included the labor costs for program staff, materials, and administrative overhead. Low, medium, and high cost estimates for programs providing services to each of the three risk groups were developed. To complete Table 3.1, the low cost estimates were assigned to the optimistic scenario, high cost estimates to the pessimistic scenario, and medium cost estimates to the base case scenario.

Note that we are not claiming that inexpensive programs are actually more effective than expensive programs. Rather, we have developed a range of scenarios reflecting optimistic, base, and pessimistic assumptions regarding HIV prevention. The optimistic scenario has high-end effectiveness estimates combined with low costs, while the pessimistic scenario has low-end effectiveness estimates combined with high costs. Nor are we claiming that the most expensive programs are least effective, or that the most effective programs are least expensive. Rather, the idea was to cover a wide range of possibilities with a very small number of scenarios. Some of the types of interventions used to construct the scenarios for the analysis include: individual risk reduction education, group counseling and skills training, community-level interventions in housing projects, identification and training of peer leaders to endorse and recommend safer-sex practices, counseling and HIV testing, partner notification, drug treatment, the provision of bleach for needle cleaning, needle exchange, and syringe access (e.g., via pharmacies).[1]

ALLOCATING RESOURCES FOR HIV PREVENTION

Following the development of these data, the Committee employed a standard model to allocate resources in order to maximize the number of infections averted. The input quantities r_{ij} and n_{ij} were obtained from Holmberg's 1996 study (see above). The input quantities c_j, f_j, and e_j are all summarized in Table 3.1. The input parameter B, the budget, is varied in the analysis from $0 to $1 billion. The decision variables x_{ij} were optimally determined via the linear program. Once determined, the number of infections averted follows. The mathematical statement of this model is presented below:

---

[1]For a complete list of interventions used in the analysis, see references at the end of this appendix.

Let:

x_{ij} = \$ allocated for programs targeting risk group j in state i
c_j = cost per program participant in programs for risk group j
e_j = % reduction in the rate of new HIV infections for those in programs for risk group j
f_j = maximum % of population reachable in risk group j
r_{ij} = annual number of new HIV infections in risk group j, state i
n_{ij} = number of person in risk group j, state i
B = HIV prevention budget

Any proposed allocation of funds corresponds to specifying numerical values for the variables x_{ij} defined above. Estimating the number of infections averted that corresponds to a proposed funding allocation to programs for risk group j in state i requires four computational steps:

(i) First, divide allocated amounts by per capita program costs to obtain the number of persons that could be reached:

The number of persons reached with programs in j, state $i = \dfrac{x_{ij}}{c_j}$.

(ii) Second, compare the result of (i) to the maximum number of persons who can be reached to determine the actual number reached:

The actual number of persons reached equals the minimum of $\dfrac{x_{ij}}{c_j}$ and $n_{ij}f_j$.

(iii) Third, apply the percentage reductions in the rate of new infections to the appropriate HIV incidence base rate to obtain the annual number of new HIV infections averted per program participant:

The number of HIV infections averted per program participant equals

$\dfrac{r_{ij}}{n_{ij}} \times e_j$.

(iv) Fourth, multiply the number of program participants [from (ii)] by the number of HIV infections averted per program participant [from (iii)] to obtain the total number of infections averted.

The number of infections prevented with programs in group j, state i
= the number reached × rate of new infections × % reduction

$$= \ \min\left(\frac{x_{ij}}{c_j}, n_{ij}f_j\right) \times \frac{r_{ij}}{n_{ij}} \times e_j.$$

Cumulating over all locations and risk groups leads to an estimate of the total number of infections prevented under any given funding allocation. We have used the four-step procedure above to estimate the effectiveness of proportional allocation schemes in the examples discussed in Chapter 3 by choosing the funding amounts x_{ij} to be proportional to the rates of new infection r_{ij} in the Holmberg (1996) data set.

To determine the allocation scheme that prevents as many infections as possible subject to a budget constraint requires selecting the funding amounts x_{ij} that solve the following linear program:

$$\max \sum_i \sum_j \frac{x_{ij}}{c_j} \times \frac{r_{ij}}{n_{ij}} \times e_j$$

subject to:

$$\frac{x_{ij}}{c_j} \le f_j n_{ij} \text{ for all } i, j$$

$$\sum_i \sum_j x_{ij} \le B$$

$$x_{ij} \ge 0 \text{ for all } i, j$$

In words, this formula says that funds should be allocated to programs for different risk groups in different states so as to maximize the number of HIV infections prevented. The constraints state: that the number of persons reached in any risk group and in any state cannot exceed the maximum number that can be reached; that the entire amount of money allocated cannot exceed the total HIV prevention budget; and that the amounts allocated toward any risk group in any state are nonnegative. For related technical literature describing the application of such models to HIV prevention, see Kahn (1996), Kaplan (1998), Kaplan and Pollack (1998), Paltiel and Stinnett (1998), and Richter, Brandeau and Owens (1999). For a didactic discussion of economic evaluation as it applies to HIV prevention, see Kaplan (1998).

SPECIFIC REFERENCES USED IN DEVELOPING MODEL SCENARIOS FOR HIV PREVENTION

Belcher L, Kalichman S, Topping M, Smith S, Emshoff J, Norris F, Nurss J. 1998. A randomized trial of a brief HIV risk reduction counseling intervention for women. *Journal of Consulting and Clinical Psychology* 66(5):856–861.

Carey MP, Maisto SA, Kalichman SC, Forsyth AD, Wright EM, Johnson BT. 1997. Enhancing motivation to reduce the risk of HIV infection for economically disadvantaged urban women. *Journal of Consulting and Clinical Psychology* 65(4):531–541.

Choi KH, Lew S, Vittinghoff E, Catania JA, Barrett DC, Coates TJ. 1996. The efficacy of brief group counseling in HIV risk reduction among homosexual Asian and Pacific Islander men. *AIDS* 10(1):81–87.

DiClemente RJ and Wingood GM. 1995. A randomized controlled trial of an HIV sexual risk-reduction intervention for young African-American women. *Journal of the American Medical Association* 274(16):1271–1276.

Hobfoll SE, Jackson AP, Lavin J, Britton PJ, Shepherd JB. 1994. Reducing inner-city women's AIDS risk activities: a study of single, pregnant women. *Health Psychology* 13(5):397–403.

Holtgrave DR (Ed.). 1998. *Handbook of Economic Evaluation of HIV Prevention Programs*. New York: Plenum Press.

Holtgrave DR and Kelly JA. 1996. Preventing HIV/AIDS among high-risk urban women: The cost-effectiveness of a behavioral group intervention. *American Journal of Public Health* 86(10):1442–1445.

Ickovics JR, Morrill AC, Beren SE, Walsh U, Rodin J. 1994. Limited effects of HIV counseling and testing for women. A prospective study of behavioral and psychological consequences. *Journal of the American Medical Association* 272(6):443–448.

Kahn JG. 1998. Economic Evaluation of Primary HIV Prevention in Injection Drug Users. In Holtgrave DR, (Ed.), *Handbook of Economic Evaluation of HIV Prevention Programs*. New York: Plenum Press. Pp. 45–62.

Kegeles SM, Hays RB, Coates TJ. 1996. The Mpowerment Project: A community-level HIV prevention intervention for young gay men. *American Journal of Public Health* 86(8 Pt 1):1129–1136.

Kegeles SM, Hays RB, Pollack LM, Coates TJ. 1999. Mobilizing young gay and bisexual men for HIV prevention: A two-community study. *AIDS* 13(13):1753–1762.

Kelly JA, Murphy DA, Sikkema KJ, McAuliffe TL, Roffman RA, Solomon LJ, Winett RA, Kalichman SC. 1997. Randomised, controlled, community-level HIV-prevention intervention for sexual-risk behaviour among homosexual men in U.S. cities. Community HIV Prevention Research Collaborative. *Lancet* 350(9090):1500–1505.

Kelly JA, Murphy DA, Washington CD, Wilson TS, Koob JJ, Davis DR, Ledezma G, Davantes B. 1994. The effects of HIV/AIDS intervention groups for high-risk women in urban clinics. *American Journal of Public Health* 84(12):1918–1922.

Kelly JA, St. Lawrence JS, Betts R, Brasfield TL, Hood HV. 1990. A skills-training group intervention model to assist persons in reducing risk behaviors for HIV infection. *AIDS Education and Prevention* 2(1):24–35.

Kelly JA, St. Lawrence JS, Diaz YE, Stevenson LY, Hauth AC, Brasfield TL, Kalichman SC, Smith JE, Andrew ME. 1991. HIV risk behavior reduction following intervention with key opinion leaders of population: An experimental analysis. *American Journal of Public Health* 81(2):168–171.

Kelly JA, St. Lawrence JS, Hood HV, Brasfield TL. 1989. Behavioral intervention to reduce AIDS risk activities. *Journal of Consulting and Clinical Psychology* 57(1):60–67.

Kelly JA, St. Lawrence JS, Stevenson LY, Hauth AC, Kalichman SC, Diaz YE, Brasfield TL, Koob JJ, Morgan MG. 1992. Community AIDS/HIV risk reduction: the effects of endorsements by popular people in three cities. *American Journal of Public Health* 82(11):1483–1489.

Peterson JL, Coates TJ, Catania J, Hauck WW, Acree M, Daigle D, Hillard B, Middleton L, Hearst N. 1996. Evaluation of an HIV risk reduction intervention among African-American homosexual and bisexual men. *AIDS* 10(3):319–325.

Pinkerton SD, Holtgrave DR, DiFranceisco WJ, Stevenson LY, Kelly JA. 1998. Cost-effectiveness of a community-level HIV risk reduction intervention. *American Journal of Public Health* 88(8):1239–1242.

Pinkerton SD, Holtgrave DR, Valdiserri RO. 1997. Cost-effectiveness of HIV-prevention skills training for men who have sex with men. *AIDS* 11(3):347–357.

Richter A, Brandeau ML, Owens DK. 1999. An analysis of optimal resource allocation for prevention of infection with human immunodeficiency virus (HIV) in injection drug users and non-users. *Medical Decision Making* 19(2):167–179.

Shain R, Piper J, Newton E, Perdue S, Ramos R, Champion J, Guerra F. 1999. A randomized controlled trail of a behavioral intervention to prevent sexually transmitted disease among minority women. *New England Journal of Medicine* 340(2):93–100.

Sikkema KJ, Kelly JA, Winett RA, Solomon LJ, Cargill VA, Roffman RA, McAuliffe TL, Heckman TG, Anderson EA, Wagstaff DA, Norman AD, Perry MJ, Crumble DA, Mercer MB. 2000. Outcomes of a randomized community-level HIV prevention intervention for women living in 18 low-income housing developments. *American Journal of Public Health* 90(1):57–63.

Stein JA, Nyamathi A, Kingston R. 1997. Change in AIDS risk behaviors among impoverished minority women after a community-based cognitive behavioral outreach program. *Journal of Community Psychology* 25:519–533.

Valdiserri RO, Lyter DW, Leviton LC, Callahan CM, Kingsley LA, Rinaldo CR. 1989. AIDS prevention in homosexual and bisexual men: Results of a randomized trial evaluating two risk reduction interventions. *AIDS* 3(1):21–26.

REFERENCES

Anderson RM and May RM. 1991. *Infectious Diseases of Humans: Dynamics and Control*. Oxford University Press: Oxford, England.

Gorsky RD. 1996. A method to measure the costs of counseling for HIV prevention. *Public Health Reports* 111(Suppl 1):115–122.

Holmberg SD. 1996. The estimated prevalence and incidence of HIV in 96 large U.S. metropolitan areas. *American Journal of Public Health* 86:642–654.

Holtgrave DR (Ed.). 1998. *Handbook of Economic Evaluation of HIV Prevention Programs*. New York: Plenum Press.

Kahn JG. 1996. The cost-effectiveness of HIV prevention targeting: How much more bang for the buck? *American Journal of Public Health*. 86:1709–1712.

Kaplan EH. 1998. Economic Evaluation and HIV Prevention Community Planning—A Policy Analyst's Perspective. In Holtgrave DR (Ed.), *Handbook of Economic Evaluation of HIV Prevention Programs*. New York: Plenum Press. Pp. 177–193.

Kaplan EH and Pollack H. 1998. Allocating HIV prevention resources. *Socio-Economic Planning Sciences* 32:257–263.

Paltiel AD and Stinnett AA. 1998. Resource allocation and the funding of HIV prevention. In Holtgrave DR (Ed.), *Handbook of Economic Evaluation of HIV Prevention Programs*. New York: Plenum Press.

Richter A, Brandeau ML, Owens DL. 1999. An analysis of optimal resource allocation for prevention of infection with human immunodeficiency virus (HIV) infection in drug users. *Medical Decision Making* 19(2):167–179.

E

Data Gathering Activities

Tom Burroughs

I. COMMUNITY PLANNING LEADERSHIP SUMMIT

On March 29, 2000, members of the IOM Committee attended the Community Planning Leadership Summit in Los Angeles, CA, to hear invited presentations and to conduct informal meetings with individuals involved in the HIV/AIDS community planning process at the federal, state, and local levels. Among the central topics discussed, the participants examined what progress has been made in HIV/AIDS prevention, what barriers still hinder prevention efforts, and what steps are needed to help overcome those barriers. Although this review cannot cover all of the issues discussed, the following descriptions cover some representative samples of the observations.

Community planning, as an official at the Centers for Disease Control and Prevention (CDC) noted, should be built on three basic principles. The first is that participation by a broad range of community members— or "community voices"—is essential. The second is that funding for HIV/ AIDS prevention should try to "get ahead" of the epidemic, rather than follow outbreaks of infection. The third is that interventions should be based on sound science and public health practice.

Although efforts are being made to expand the range of "community voices" participating in planning groups, some populations remain relatively underrepresented, according to the participants. For example, African American and Latino populations often are not adequately represented, given that these racial/ethic groups are particularly hard hit by

HIV/AIDS, especially in large metropolitan areas. Many participants also noted the importance of maintaining representation on planning groups by people living with HIV/AIDS and by people whose lives are significantly but indirectly affected by HIV/AIDS, such as the family members of infected individuals.

In trying to keep funding for prevention abreast of changes in the epidemic, many participants noted that major challenges remain in serving men who have sex with men, as well as injection drug users. Men from racial and ethnic minority groups, including gay men, bisexual men, and men who do not identify themselves with either of these groups, are of particular concern, as they now comprise a majority of the HIV/AIDS cases among men who have sex with men. Some participants said that heterosexual women, particularly women from racial and ethnic minority groups, who now represent the largest proportion of women impacted by HIV/AIDS, are in need of increased attention as well. In this regard, participants called for more research to be devoted to developing prevention methods that women themselves can control, such as microbicides. Increased prevention efforts also should be targeted at young people, many of whom are sexually active and, because they came of age after the first flourish of HIV/AIDS prevention activities, may not have gained adequate knowledge of risk behaviors and methods to reduce those risks.

In addition, participants noted that as new treatments are becoming available, more people are living with HIV/AIDS, and thus it is becoming increasingly important to target interventions to reach HIV-infected individuals. In some communities, the participants reported, growing numbers of infected individuals apparently are resuming high risk behaviors that hold potential for spreading the epidemic. Advances in treatment are having another effect as well, according to some participants, who noted their worry that more and more policymakers, from the federal to the local level, seem to be shifting both their concern and their budget priorities, away from prevention and toward treatment-only programs.

There was some disagreement about whether prevention interventions being used today are indeed based on the latest scientific evidence. Federal officials generally maintained that the majority of prevention programs being implemented incorporate methods that many observers view as effective. Some representatives of state agencies and private groups, however, suggested that in some communities, both the planning process and intervention efforts are often "more gut-based than evidence-based," as one participant said. All participants agreed that more attention should be directed at program evaluation in order to document—in a variety of communities, using a variety of interventions, and focusing on a variety of at-risk populations—which prevention methods work best under particular conditions. In this regard, some participants pointed out the need to evaluate interventions conducted in rural areas, where conditions often are greatly different than in metropolitan areas with higher concentrations of at-risk individuals, and where local experience offers little guidance for success. Evaluation also should be directed at determining the cost-effectiveness of various interventions, as such information generally is lacking. As one participant from a city HIV/AIDS prevention office reported, "We make many of our program decisions based on 'cost and assumption' of effectiveness, rather than on solid evidence of actual cost and effectiveness." Such evaluation efforts, participants added, should incorporate improved systems of data collection and should involve longer-term follow-up that typically is used today.

One major area of agreement among participants is that there must be a greater level of coordination and cooperation in all aspects of HIV/AIDS prevention, from the funding and planning of programs to their implementation and evaluation in specific communities. Many participants from state and private groups agreed, as one participant noted, that "the HIV prevention system is poorly coordinated and accounted for within and across government agencies."

At the federal level, a participant from a national AIDS organization called for more coordination among the Health Resources and Services Administration (HRSA), the Department of Health and Human Services (DHHS), the National Institutes of Health (NIH), and the CDC in developing programs that address multiple issues related to prevention. A representative of a state AIDS agency added that "CDC and HRSA must do a much better job of working with each other to identify prevention goals." In particular, there was a strong call, endorsed by numerous participants, for more coordination between federal and state agencies to ensure that local community planning groups get the resources they are requesting to improve prevention efforts. Several participants also called for establishing a single point of contact for federal and state funding to streamline the process and ensure that all state and local groups, both public and private, have equitable access to "the system."

Coordination of both funding and programs needs to be improved at the state and local levels as well. "We sometimes have two agencies funding programs in the same locations, and neither the funders nor the groups carrying out the interventions really know what the other project is about," according to a representative of one state agency. Another participant from a city HIV/AIDS group noted that the community planning process has become "essentially disconnected" from the health department. Participants also said there should be better communication and interaction among researchers studying some aspect of HIV/AIDS prevention in a particular community and those groups or individuals who actually are conducting the prevention. "Too often, researchers come in, gather the data they want, and then leave," noted one local HIV/AIDS representative. "We never hear from them again about what they learned or how we might benefit. They seem to be focused mostly on publishing the results in some scientific journal."

Participants noted that interventions should be targeted increasingly at groups of people who are at highest risk of HIV/AIDS. These groups often vary by region, state, community, or even, as has been found in many cases, on a block-by-block basis. Planning groups should make identifying these at-risk populations a priority. As one participant from a state agency reported, "We can't simply rely on what we 'know to be true' from national statistics, or on what we have read about regarding other communities, because these data often turn out to be untrue or outdated for our particular community. We've got to find out who faces the highest risks in our own local areas."

Prevention efforts then should be conducted in a consistent, on-going, and nonintrusive manner. Intervention services should be made available in the neighborhoods where high risk individuals live, congregate, procure drugs, or engage in sex trade, and the services should be readily available at the times when recipients most need them. Interventions should be culturally appropriate and, in some cases, language specific. Culture in this case includes not only ethic and racial considerations, but also the culture of the specific community in which at-risk individuals live or socialize. Said one representative of a national AIDS organization: "Consider just gay men, for example. There's a difference in the strategies that need to be used to reach men in the rural south, or men of color living in a New York ghetto, or men living in Latino communities. These men all have different social and cultural contexts, and we need to develop ways to reach each of these populations that will have the greatest impact in changing their behaviors."

One major challenge in reaching many target populations, especially those often marginalized by society, is the need to develop a sense of trust between the service providers and service recipients. Many of these populations, said the participants, have developed a profound lack of trust in official systems. "Often, this mistrust is well rooted in their life experiences," noted a representative of a city HIV/AIDS group. "In too many cases, official systems—from the public health system to the legal system to public service systems—have by and large not recognized or valued their fragile life situations." Developing interventions that foster an individual's long-term engagement will be key in turning around this distrust and making prevention efforts seem safer and more user-friendly to increasing numbers of people now out of reach of conventional public and private programs.

To help them in developing and implementing prevention programs, many communities need increased technical assistance from federal and state agencies, as well as private organizations, that have experience in this area. Some participants noted that this is a particular need among groups working in racial and ethnic minority communities, where, until recently, attention to and funding for HIV/AIDS programs has been limited. A representative of one federally supported organization that provides such services defined technical assistance as the provision of direct or indirect support to increase the skills of individuals and/or groups to carry out programmatic and management responsibilities with respect to HIV/AIDS prevention. Help is available in such areas as community planning, use of epidemiological data for decision-making, assessment of local needs, and evaluation of intervention effectiveness. The goal is to help communities develop their own capacity to assess their needs, coordinate the intervention from beginning to end, and assess the outcomes. However, some participants noted that current federally funded technical assistance programs work in only a piecemeal way. This creates a system of technical assistance by which communities and organizations get isolated help with one planning component area, such as data collection or social and behavioral science theory. But what is lacking is integrated technical assistance that shows how each of these components is interconnected.

It is becoming increasingly important that HIV/AIDS prevention and treatment programs be offered in conjunction with a range of other health and social services, many participants noted. Such integration will provide an increased number of avenues for reaching at-risk individuals. Primary care facilities, drug treatment centers, sexually transmitted diseases clinics, and mental health centers all should have the capacity to deliver HIV/AIDS prevention services. Building this capacity in many cases will require investing more resources to equip the facilities and to train staff. But this integrated approach offers the potential to draw more infected and at-risk individuals into the general health care and social services systems, where they can receive a wide range of services to help them meet the numerous pressing needs they often face in their everyday lives.

Some methods of HIV/AIDS intervention have proved to be socially or politically controversial, and many participants called on public agencies and public health officials to argue for their incorporation in comprehensive prevention campaigns. For example, numerous participants said there is ample scientific evidence that needle exchange and needle cleaning programs are effective in reducing the incidence of HIV/AIDS among injection drug users and their sexual partners, and that such programs do not result in an increase in illegal drug use. "We have the capacity to reduce effectively HIV transmission among injection-drug users, but we don't have the political will to provide the resources so these strategies can be implemented on a nationwide basis," one representative of a national HIV/AIDS organization maintained. "By that, I mean there is no political will to lift the ban on using federal funds for needle-exchange programs." Some states have gone ahead with such programs without federal support, and several representatives from state agencies reported that their programs have indeed proved successful. Some of these representatives, however, expressed worry over stories they have heard about moves within the federal government to block funding for all HIV/AIDS treatment and prevention to states that support their own needle exchange programs. Community programs that include the distribution of condoms, as well as school programs that describe HIV/AIDS prevention measures other than abstinence, also have come under fire in some locations. Participants said they want public policymakers to strongly endorse the importance of providing condoms in prevention programs, and to encourage local school districts to implement comprehensive sex education and condom availability in their health programs. As one participant concluded, "Leadership is needed in making the case, to the public and to policy makers, that sanctioning interventions to prevent HIV infection is not equivalent to sanctioning the behaviors that transmit the disease."

II. REQUEST FOR PUBLIC COMMENT

The IOM Committee issued a request for public comment to obtain input on issues relating to state and local HIV/AIDS prevention efforts. The request, which was posted on the project Web site, asked for responses to questions in six general areas: data needs, technical assistance, translation of prevention research into practice, program evaluation, coordination and implementation of programs, and opportunities and barriers. The Committee received 32 responses from individuals and organizations in 19 states and Washington, D.C. Comments were submitted by a variety of groups, including state health departments, local health departments, and capacity-building organizations, as well as by members of the general public. Although this review cannot cover all of the comments submitted, the following descriptions cover some representative samples of the observations.

Data Needs

Numerous respondents cited the need for the federal government to create a national name-based HIV/AIDS surveillance system. "This is necessary to understand the current burden and epidemiological profile of the disease and to appropriately allocate funds and target interventions," noted a state HIV/AIDS program official. Respondents also noted the need to increase behavioral surveillance in order to better analyze patterns in risk behavior, to expand data collection in rural areas, and to improve data collection on the incidence and prevalence of HIV/AIDS in federal and state correctional institutions. In addition, many respondents said that, at the local level, community planning groups need better data to pinpoint the populations at greatest risk for new HIV infections and to identify the service needs of persons living with HIV/AIDS. Local groups also need to receive from the federal government specific information and techniques on how to prioritize target populations from epidemiologic profiles.

As one caveat regarding the need for expanded data collection, a state agency representative made the following request: "Do not ask states to institute complex prevention data and reporting systems that focus primarily on the need of the federal government to justify prevention. This sometimes makes it difficult to focus on real prevention and evaluation data needs."

Technical Assistance

Federal and state agencies should better coordinate their technical assistance efforts, to minimize overlap in funding and data gathering and to ensure that all prevention programs have adequate infrastructure to carry out their activities. "There is significant duplication of effort between the technical assistance efforts of the Centers for Disease Control and Prevention (CDC) and the Health Resources and Services Administration (HRSA)," said a former state HIV/AIDS program official. "While each agency should have the capacity to deliver technical assistance on request of its grantees, such assistance should be coordinated so that prevention and care groups locally benefit."

Respondents also noted that not enough attention currently is paid to the value of peer-to-peer technical assistance. "One jurisdiction can be very helpful to another, and often this will be more effective than having a federal employee trying to figure out what a jurisdiction needs, especially without having direct experience," reported a state HIV/AIDS program official. Some respondents also called for technical assistance that is more practical than theoretical or organizational in nature. "For example, with outreach, we want to learn exactly where to go, at what time, what to bring, what to wear, how to act, what to say in this situation or that situation, what to do with this person or that person, and so on," one foundation official said. "We want real hands-on help in how to better work with our clients in our local environment, not more theories and generalizations of application."

Translation of Prevention Research into Practice

Many respondents suggested that the translation of prevention research into practice often has been too slow. Various suggestions were offered to speed up this process. For example, CDC was called on to establish an interactive Web site that would enable its grantees and others to rapidly exchange information about prevention initiatives.

Respondents from some community groups also reported that they are having difficulty obtaining up-to-date information about intervention programs and their effectiveness. To help overcome such problems, a state HIV/AIDS program official suggested that research findings from federally supported studies should be disseminated in a timely manner and in a format that is easily accessible by a variety of audiences. "Guidelines for application to intervention development and/or refinement should accompany the research findings," the respondent added. Other program representatives suggested that, in order to facilitate rapid dissemination of research findings, federal agencies should be encouraged to use multiple technologies, including Internet technologies and satellite teleconferences.

Few community-based organizations have the staff or resource capability to employ or retain behavioral or social scientists to conduct HIV/AIDS prevention research, according to respondents. On the other hand, there are few incentives for researchers to form collaborative partnerships with community-based organizations that go beyond a specific research project. As a result, there is often a "disconnect" between research and program implementation. One proposed solution is that research funding should promote such collaboration and partnership to build community capacity so that its prevention efforts not only benefit at-risk individuals but also contribute to HIV/AIDS prevention science.

Program Evaluation

Evaluating how well interventions work has been a key "missing link" in prevention efforts. As one state HIV/AIDS program official said, "It is unfortunate that we are just now beginning to evaluate our prevention programs systematically, under a common guidance, some 12 to 13 years into federal funding of these programs. Any new initiatives required by CDC should learn from this and build an evaluation component into new funding initiatives and their program requirements."

CDC also was called on to provide local jurisdictions with more guidance on how to conduct cost-effectiveness studies.

Program evaluation can be especially difficult for states that receive only minimal funding for HIV/AIDS prevention. "We need funds for hardware, software, and technical assistance to set up the computer-based data collection systems that will assist us in outcome evaluations," reported one university researcher working with the state health department.

Some respondents added that the term "evaluation" itself needs to be better defined, in order to ensure consistency in evaluations conducted by different types of groups working at various locations.

Coordination and Implementation of Programs

Many respondents called for improved coordination of all aspects of HIV/AIDS prevention, from the funding and planning of programs to their implementation and evaluation in specific communities. Lack of coordination among federal agencies, such as CDC and HRSA, is pinpointed as the cause of "red tape" that slows down the progress of state and local organizations. Translation of behavioral or social science also has been greatly hampered by lack of coordination among federal agencies engaged in research and those supporting prevention and care services. "It is critical that research agendas be developed collaboratively among federal agencies to assure that research activities clearly address priority needs related to program development and support, and that findings are applied to program refinement in a timely manner," noted a state HIV/AIDS program official.

There also needs to be better coordination between groups or facilities that provide HIV/AIDS prevention and facilities that provide other health-related services, such as primary care clinics, drug treatment centers, sexually transmitted diseases clinics, and mental health centers. "It is very difficult to put prevention interventions into place for only HIV/AIDS clients and to ignore the need to provide similar messages and programs for other sexually transmitted diseases," a state HIV/AIDS program official said.

In terms of implementing prevention programs, respondents agreed that one size does not fit all. Rather, interventions should be tailored to specific needs, and programs need to be culturally relevant and, in many cases, language specific in order to reach targeted at-risk populations. Intervention services also should be made available in areas where high-risk individuals live or socialize, and the services should be readily available at the times when recipients most need them.

Respondents also pointed to some special needs. For example, federal and state agencies should recognize and address the impact of rural cultural differences on HIV/AIDS prevention efforts. "These differences must be considered in development and funding of prevention interventions," said one state HIV/AIDS program official, and respondents called for one of these agencies to develop a guide or summary document regarding effective interventions in rural areas. In addition, agencies need to learn more about how to serve specific subpopulations—including vision-impaired or hearing-impaired individuals, women who are injection-drug users, and adolescent sex workers—who typically have not been targeted for intervention. "Individuals with special needs often lack sufficient training or educational literature that address those specific needs," a state HIV/AIDS program official noted. "For example, how do you demonstrate condom use to an individual who is blind or to someone who is mentally challenged?"

Opportunities and Barriers

Many respondents reported that their greatest barrier continues to be a shortage of financial resources to implement prevention programs. "Our state's planning activities are very strong, but community members become frustrated when they want to implement local plans but don't have sufficient resources to do so," noted one state HIV/AIDS program official.

Respondents also noted that there appears to be growing complacency among funders, policymakers, the media, and even many community members about HIV/AIDS prevention, while at the same time there continues to be a growing sentiment among policymakers that HIV/AIDS is treated preferentially, receiving a disproportionate among of funding and attention compared with other health issues. These respondents went on to say that renewed leadership is required, at the national, state, and local levels, to re-engage governmental and nongovernmental support for HIV/AIDS prevention programs.

Among the various opportunities cited, respondents wanted federal and state agencies to expand mass media HIV/AIDS prevention education messages that support local efforts to educate the public on the entire continuum of risk reduction and the level of risk associated with specific behaviors. These messages should be nonjudgmental but communicate that HIV/AIDS is still a dangerous and ultimately fatal disease. Respondents also suggested that in many racial and ethnic minority communities, ethnic media have been greatly underutilized. Such media, especially ethnic radio, offer lower cost ways to reach target populations.

In the educational arena, many respondents called for federal and state agencies to support implementation of classroom instruction on the transmission and prevention of sexually transmitted diseases, including HIV/AIDS. The federal government, they said, should reconsider its prohibition against funding school programs that discuss prevention strategies other than abstinence. "This often forces schools to choose between politically correct abstinence and effective comprehensive skills-based instruction." One parent, however, suggested that it is appropriate that schools offer programs that discuss only abstinence, arguing that condoms are known to fail and that young people are best counseled to save sex until marriage.

To address the disproportionate impact of disease in racial and ethnic minority communities, the federal government should increase collaboration among agencies working on HIV/AIDS prevention and the Office of Minority Health. In particular, the government should fund demonstration projects to provide a continuum of health-related services within minority communities. This broader-brush approach would affect many diseases and events—including stroke, heart attack, diabetes, and homicide—along with decreasing the incidence of HIV/AIDS.

To foster HIV/AIDS prevention among injection drug users, federal and state agencies should increase their funding in order to increase the number of "treatment slots" in substance abuse programs. Some respondents noted that there is, in particular, a shortage of funding slots for special populations (for example, women with children, HIV-infected persons with mental illness, immigrants, and the formerly incarcerated). Federal and state agencies also should expand training provided to substance abuse prevention and treatment providers regarding basic information on HIV/AIDS and effective prevention strategies. Many respondents also suggested that the federal government should lift its restrictions on the use of federal resources for needle exchange programs. "My state conducts syringe exchange without using federal funding, but our budget currently limits how far we can integrate this program into the whole of HIV prevention," said one public health official. "CDC must continue to make progress on addressing HIV infection among injection drug users by asserting that syringe exchange programs are a high-priority intervention that needs to become fully funded."

III. SITE VISITS TO STATE HEALTH DEPARTMENTS

During the course of the study, four Committee members conducted interviews with officials working in state and city health departments. Two of these departments are located in the northeastern United States, one in the mid-Atlantic region, and one in the northwest region. These visits were considered data-gathering sessions and were intended to inform the Committee with regard to prevention activities at the state and local level.

The conversations were constructed around seven primary questions the Committee members were asked to address. The issues that were covered included: HIV prevention strategies, data needs, technical assistance, program evaluation, potential collaborations, opportunities, and barriers.

General Comments

- Officials stated that CDC does not seem to care what the community thinks when it comes to their strategic plan.
- Officials expressed concern about the lack of coordination within CDC itself.
- It is believed that the CDC has "little in house behavioral science expertise."
- The CDC won't support good existing programs (it's more likely to provide money for new programs), and this undercuts the notion of doing evaluations.
- There's a lack of communication between CDC and local organizations (e.g., state health departments) when it comes to prevention efforts.
- The health departments reported trying to get the Community Planning Groups (CPGs) to look at cost-effectiveness three years ago, but due to a lack of systematic information about cost-effectiveness across all prevention programs, it could not be used as a criterion.

How do you prioritize and select HIV prevention strategies to implement in your state (or city)?

- Prioritize based on: demonstrated need, intervention effectiveness, and cost analysis.
- Prioritize using HIV/AIDS epidemiological data (mainly AIDS cases), service delivery data (where are people going for care), Medicaid data, recommendations from CPGs, cost-effectiveness data, and proven interventions.
- The prevention plan is written by the Community Planning Group according to CDC guidelines, which require needs be based on criteria such as epidemiological profiles and needs assessments. The department contracts with various agencies to carry out different parts of the plan.
- One health department reported that priorities are sometimes set using data that the state provides but, at other times, are based on anecdotes or other issues that the department values intrinsically. "People believe what they want to believe regardless of the data."

What additional information would be most helpful to you in planning, implementing, or monitoring HIV prevention programs in your state (or city)?

- Would like to see better HIV incidence or prevalence data, STD data, drug use data, and youth behavioral risk data, and more information about the mental health needs and issues of targeted populations.
- "Serosurvey information on new infections would be most helpful . . . prevalence information in different populations would be helpful."
- Develop methods to go from research to real-life interventions.
- It was noted that there is a strong need for evaluation funds, since funds for evaluation are currently coming from service funds.
- Would like to see realistic information on the efficacy of programs.

What additional types of technical assistance does your state (or city) need from the federal government to better support HIV prevention activities?

- Would like to see realistic technical assistance on cost-effectiveness.
- National conferences should be held (like the one CDC held in August of 1999) in order to bridge the gap between reality and research.
- Funds for more collaborative projects involving community based organizations, health departments, and HIV prevention researchers.
- Tailored models of intervention (CDC's top down model of technology transfer is inadequate).

How do you evaluate whether HIV prevention programs in your state (or city) are working?

- Review epidemiological data, solicitation of community views and perspectives, assessment of referrals and linkages to care, cost effectiveness, monitor youth behavioral risk data, drug use and behavior (i.e., syringe sharing), and mental health data.

Are there potential new partnerships or alliances that you would like the health departments to pursue related to HIV prevention efforts? What role do you envision these partners having?

- Would like to see more money for collaborative projects involving community based organizations (CBOs), health departments, and HIV prevention researchers.
- Faith communities to help advance HIV prevention, especially among racial and ethnic minority communities.
- Partnerships with HIV/AIDS prevention research centers.
- Center for AIDS Prevention Studies, UCSF to strengthen intervention, strategies, technology diffusion, and advance community planning.

What are the most significant barriers that you encounter to planning or implementing effective HIV prevention programs in your state (or city)?

- While we know a lot about effective invention strategies, there are still political barriers to implementing these strategies (e.g., needle exchange, condom distribution, comprehensive sex education).
- There's a need for cost-effectiveness data (rating system), national summaries about effectiveness, technical assistance that pays attention to cultural competence, better prevalence/incidence data, and guidance on cost/unit calculations.
- There is a lack of a strong federal public health initiative to address the ongoing HIV epidemic.
- The ban on use of federal funds for needle-exchange programs hinders ability to reduce HIV infection in IDUs, their sexual partners, and their children.
- Lack of capacity (financial, administrative) among community-based organizations is an ongoing problem.
- Populations most strongly effected by HIV/AIDS are viewed as expendable.
- Confidentiality concerns: there is an eroding of confidentiality protections (e.g., HIV name reporting, trends toward criminalization).

What are the most significant, unrealized opportunities for improved HIV prevention in your state (or city)?

- Would like to create more partnerships with academic institutions.
- Would like to see more collaboration between prevention programs and care programs for HIV-infected individuals.

F

Agendas for
Public Committee Meetings

FIRST MEETING

January 24, 2000
National Academies Building, Washington, D.C.

Welcome and Introductions
IOM Committee
Liaison Panel
Other guests

Presentation of the Charge to the Committee by Sponsoring Agency
Ronald Valdiserri, M.D., M.P.H.
Deputy Director, National Center for HIV, STD, TB Prevention, Centers for Disease Control and Prevention

Presentations from the CDC Advisory Committee on HIV and STD Prevention
HIV Prevention Research
King Holmes, M.D., Ph.D.
Director, Center for AIDS and STD, University of Washington, Seattle

HIV Prevention Policy
Dorothy Mann
Executive Director, Southeastern Pennsylvania Family Planning Council, Philadelphia

HIV Prevention and Service Delivery Programs
Jean McGuire, Ph.D.
Director, AIDS Bureau, Massachusetts Department of Public Health, Boston

Remarks by CDC Director
Jeffrey Koplan, M.D., M.P.H.
Director, Centers for Disease Control and Prevention

Centers for Disease Control and Prevention's HIV Prevention Programs
Helene Gayle, M.D., M.P.H.
Director, National Center for HIV, STD, TB Prevention, Centers for Disease Control and Prevention

HIV Prevention Research at the National Institutes of Health
Neal Nathanson, M.D.
Director, Office of AIDS Research, National Institutes of Health

Judith Auerbach, Ph.D.
Prevention Science Coordinator and Behavioral and Social Science Coordinator, Office of AIDS Research, National Institutes of Health

SECOND MEETING

March 1, 2000
National Academies Building, Washington, D.C.

Welcome and Introductions
IOM Committee
Liaison Panel
Other guests

Overview of State-Level HIV Prevention Activities
Julie Scofield
Executive Director, National Alliance of State and Territorial AIDS Directors

Gloria Maki, M.S.
Executive Deputy Director, New York State AIDS Institute

HIV Prevention in Correctional Settings
Lester Wright, M.D., M.P.H.
Associate Commissioner, Chief Medical Officer, New York Department of Correctional Services

Abstinence-Only Education and Sexually Transmitted Diseases: Theory, Practice, and Evaluation of Programs Funded Under Title V
Rebecca Maynard, Ph.D
Office of Population Research, Princeton University

Opportunities for HIV Prevention in Major Urban Epicenters
Eric Goosby, M.D.
Director, Office of HIV/AIDS Policy, U.S. Department of Health and Human Services

Overview of FDA Regulatory Responsibilities in HIV Prevention
Debra Birnkrant, M.D.
Deputy Director, Division of Antiviral Drug Products, Center for Drug Evaluation and Research

William Egan, Ph.D.
Acting Director, Office of Vaccine Research and Review, Center for Biologics Evaluation and Research

Richard Klein
HIV/AIDS Program Director, Office of Special Health Issues, Office of International and Constituent Relations

Edward Tabor, M.D.
Associate Director for Medical Affairs, Office of Blood Research and Review, Center for Biologics Evaluation and Research

Integrating HIV Prevention into the Continuum of Care
Joseph O'Neill, M.D.
Associate Administrator of AIDS, HIV/AIDS Bureau, Health Resources and Services Administration

Substance Abuse and Mental Health Issues in HIV Prevention
Melvyn Haas, M.D.
Medical Director and AIDS Coordinator, Center for Mental Health Services, Substance Abuse and Mental Health Services Administration

Eric Goplerud, Ph.D.
Acting Associate Administrator, Office of Policy and Program Coordination, Substance Abuse and Mental Health Services Administration

Overview of Department of Veterans Affairs HIV Prevention Activities
Lawrence Deyton, M.S.P.H., M.D.
Director, AIDS Service, Department of Veterans Affairs

Kim Hamlett, Ph.D.
Associate Director for Prevention, AIDS Service, Department of Veterans Affairs

THIRD MEETING

April 13, 2000
The Charles Hotel, Cambridge, Massachusetts

Welcome and Introductions
IOM Committee
Liaison Panel
Other guests

Presentations by Congressional Black Caucus Initiative Crisis Response Team Phase I Cities
Rich Needle, Ph.D., M.P.H.
National Institutes of Health, RARE Methodology

Evelyn Ullah, B.S.N., M.S.W.
Director, Office of HIV/AIDS Services, Miami Crisis Response Team

David Acosta
Director, Prevention Programs and Services, The AIDS Activities Office, Philadelphia Crisis Response Team

Renee McCoy
Ethnographer, Detroit Crisis Response Team

Question-and-Answer Period

Involving People with HIV in HIV Prevention
Terje Anderson
Executive Director, National Association of People with AIDS

HIV Prevention Policy Issues
Clark Moore
Director for Policy and Communications, AIDS Alliance for Children, Youth,
    and Families

HIV Prevention for Young Women
Margaret Campbell
Board of Directors, AIDS Alliance for Children, Youth, and Families, Senior
    Community Health Educator, Wayne Wright Resource Center

Open Floor

COMMUNITY PLANNING LEADERSHIP SUMMIT

March 29–30, 2000
Wilshire Hotel, Los Angeles, California

March 29, 2000
Panel I

The Future of Community Planning
David Holtgrave, Ph.D.
Director, Division of HIV AIDS Prevention, Intervention, Research, and
    Support, Centers for Disease Control and Prevention

**The Technical Assistance Process as a Part of HIV Prevention
Community Planning**
Frank Beadle de Palomo, M.A.
Director, Center for Community-Based Health Strategies, Academy of
    Educational Development

Unmet Prevention Needs in Communities of Color
Miguelina Ileana León
Director of Government Relations and Public Policy, National Minority
    AIDS Council

**Ongoing HIV Prevention Challenges: The Washington State
Perspective**
Jack Jourden, M.D., M.P.H.
Director, Infectious Disease and Reproduction

Question-and-Answer Period with Panel I

Panel II

Community-Level Perspective of the Community Planning Group Process
A. Toni Young
San Francisco Community Co-chair

Resources Utilized by the Massachusetts Community Planning Groups for HIV Prevention Planning
Kevin Cranston
Massachusetts Department of Health

Focus Groups I and II
Thursday, March 30

G

Biographies

HARVEY V. FINEBERG, M.D., M.P.P., Ph.D. (*Cochair*), became Provost of Harvard University in 1997, following 13 years as Dean of Harvard's Faculty of Public Health. He has devoted most of his academic career to the fields of health policy and medical decision making. His past research has focused on the process of policy development and implementation, assessment of medical technology, evaluation and use of vaccines, and dissemination of medical innovations. Dr. Fineberg helped found and has served as president of the Society for Medical Decision Making and also served as consultant to the World Health Organization. As a member of the Institute of Medicine, he has chaired and served on numerous panels on health policy issues, ranging from AIDS to new medical technology. He has also served as a member of the Public Health Council of Massachusetts, as chairman of the Health Care Technology Study Section of the National Center for Health Services Research, and as president of the Association of Schools of Public Health. He is the author, coauthor, and coeditor of numerous books and articles on such diverse topics as AIDS prevention, vaccine safety and understanding risk in society. In 1988, he received the Joseph W. Mountain Prize from the Centers for Disease Control and Prevention and the Wade Hampton Frost Prize from the Epidemiology Section of the American Public Health Association. Dr. Fineberg earned his degrees from Harvard University.

JAMES TRUSSELL, Ph.D. (*Cochair*), is Professor of Economics and Public Affairs, Faculty Associate of the Office of Population Research, and Associate Dean of the Woodrow Wilson School of Public and International Affairs at Princeton University. Dr. Trussell is the author or coauthor of more than 175 scientific publications, primarily in the areas of reproductive health and demographic methodology. His recent research has been focused in three areas: emergency contraception, contraceptive failure, and the cost-effectiveness of contraception. Dr. Trussell received his Ph.D. in economics from Princeton University. Dr. Trussell currently serves as a research associate of the National Bureau of Economic Research; as a member of the board of directors of The Alan Guttmacher Institute, the NARAL Foundation, and the Association of Reproductive Health Professionals; and as a member of the Council of the International Union for the Scientific Study of Population and the technical advisory committee of Family Health International. He also serves on the editorial advisory committee of *Contraception, Family Planning Perspectives, Contraceptive Technology Update,* and the *Journal of the Australian Population Association.*

RAYMOND BAXTER, Ph.D., is Executive Vice President of The Lewin Group and heads the firm's national research, policy, and management practice. His research and consulting focus on community health, health systems reform, policy development, organizational change and strategic planning. He has worked with government and the private sector at the state, local and national level, and has over 20 years of experience in public health management, including heading the San Francisco Department of Public Health and the New York City Health and Hospitals Corporation. Dr. Baxter currently leads an evaluation of the nation's disease surveillance capacity for the Assistant Secretary of Health and Human Services. For the past four years he has assisted General Motors, Chrysler, Ford and the United Auto Workers in a national initiative to assess local health system performance and to organize collaborative planning among purchasers, providers and consumers to reduce costs and improve quality. Dr. Baxter has headed the 12-site community tracking initiative of the Center for Studying Health System Change, funded by the Robert Wood Johnson Foundation. He is completing a multiyear goal-level evaluation of the W.K. Kellogg Foundation's community health grant-making and has led evaluation initiatives for the Robert Wood Johnson Foundation, the California Endowment, the David & Lucile Packard Foundation, and the federal government. Dr. Baxter has assisted numerous public, not-for-profit and private organizations in strategic plans, reorganizations and special projects. Dr. Baxter holds a Ph.D. from the Woodrow Wilson School of Public and International Affairs at Princeton University.

WILLARD CATES, JR., M.D., M.P.H., is President of the Family Health Institute of Family Health International (FHI) in North Carolina. He received a combined M.D.-M.P.H. degree from Yale School of Medicine, and trained clinically in Internal Medicine at the University of Virginia Hospital. He is board certified in Preventive Medicine. He is currently Principal Investigator of the Leadership Core of the HIV Prevention Trials Network, funded by NIH. He also is a member of the Centers for Disease Control and Prevention (CDC) Advisory Committee on HIV and STD Prevention. Prior to joining FHI, Dr. Cates was at CDC for two decades, where he served as Director of the Division of STD/HIV Prevention for half that time. Dr. Cates is a Member of the Institute of Medicine, National Academy of Sciences, the American College of Epidemiology, and past President of the Society for Epidemiologic Research. He is coauthor of two major reproductive health textbooks, and has authored or co-authored over 400 scientific publications. He is a Visiting Professor of Epidemiology at the University of North Carolina at Chapel Hill School of Public Health, the Rollins School of Public Health at Emory University, and the University of Michigan School of Public Health.

MYRON S. COHEN, M.D., is a Professor of Medicine, Microbiology and Immunology at University of North Carolina (UNC), Chief of the Division of Infectious Diseases, and Director of the UNC Center for HIV/STDs and Infectious Diseases. Dr. Cohen is on the Board of Directors of the International Society for Sexually Transmitted Disease Research and has served on a number of advisory committees for the Centers for Disease Control and Prevention and the National Institutes of Health (NIH). Dr. Cohen is Director of the NIH Sexually Transmitted Diseases Clinical Trials Network, the UNC U.S. Agency for International Development IMPACT (AIDS Prevention) Program, and the Johns Hopkins/UNC HIVNET Program. He is chair of the NIH HIV Prevention Treatment Network Antiretroviral Working Group. He is also codirector of the UNC/NIH Fogarty Center and Associate Director of the UNC/NIH Center for AIDS Research and UNC/NIH STD Cooperative Research Center. Dr. Cohen's research interests focus on the transmission and prevention of STDs and HIV. He received his M.D. from Rush Medical College, and completed his residency in internal medicine at the University of Michigan and postdoctoral fellowship in infectious diseases at Yale University.

ANKE A. EHRHARDT, Ph.D., is the Director of the HIV Center for Clinical and Behavioral Studies at the New York State Psychiatric Institute and is a Professor of Medical Psychology in the Department of Psychiatry at Columbia University. Dr. Ehrhardt came to Columbia University from the State University of New York at Buffalo where she codirected the Program of Psychoendocrinology at Children's Hospital. She was also formerly the President of the International Academy of Sex Research. Dr.

Ehrhardt is an internationally known researcher in the field of sexual and gender development of children, adolescents, and adults. For the past 25 years, her research has included a wide range of studies on determinants of sexual risk behavior among children, adolescents, heterosexual women and men, and the gay population, and on comprehensive approaches to preventing HIV and STD infection. In recognition of this work, she was presented with the Research Award "For Excellence in Research" from the State of New York Office of Mental Health in 1990 and the Award for Distinguished Scientific Achievement for 1991, from the Society for the Scientific Study of Sex. She has more than 160 scientific publications and has co-authored several books. Dr. Ehrhardt received her Ph.D. in psychology from the University of Düsseldorf, Germany and completed a postgraduate fellowship in the Psychohormonal Research Unit at The Johns Hopkins Hospital.

BRIAN FLAY, D.Phil., is the founding director of the Prevention Research Center in the School of Public Health at the University of Illinois at Chicago, and currently serves as the Director of the Health Research and Policy Centers and Professor of Community Health Sciences and Psychology. Dr. Flay's research interests include smoking and drug abuse etiology and prevention, HIV/AIDS and violence prevention, risk-taking behaviors among adolescents, and school- and community-based interventions. Dr. Flay has served on Centers for Disease Control and Prevention committees for HIV/AIDS prevention research, and the development of comprehensive school health guidelines. He served on the Expert Panel on the Evaluation of AIDS Interventions for the Committee on AIDS Research in Behavioral, Social and Statistical Sciences of the National Academy of Sciences. He was also an advisor to OSAP/CSAP on high-risk youth, media interventions and school-based interventions. In 1993, Dr. Flay received recognition for outstanding research from the Research Council of the American School Health Association. From 1994 to 1998, Dr. Flay served on several CDC and National Institutes of Health–National Advisory Committees on prevention or behavioral research (NIMH, NIDA, NIAAA, NIAID, and NCI). Dr. Flay has published more than 140 peer-reviewed publications and 25 book chapters. He is a fellow of the Society for Behavioral Medicine and the Society for Community Research and Action and is a member of the Robert Wood Johnson Funded Research Network on the Etiology of Tobacco Dependence. Dr. Flay received his D.Phil. in Social Psychology from Waikato University in New Zealand and completed postdoctoral training in evaluation research and social psychology at Northwestern University under a Fulbright/Hays Fellowship.

LORETTA JEMMOTT, Ph.D., R.N., F.A.A.N., is Associate Professor and Director of the Center for Urban Health Research at the University of Pennsylvania School of Nursing, and holds a secondary appointment in the Graduate School of Education. Dr. Jemmott received her M.S.N. in nursing, specializing in psychiatric mental health nursing, and her Ph.D. in education, specializing in human sexuality education, from the University of Pennsylvania. Since 1987, Dr. Jemmott's research has focused on designing and testing theory-based, culturally sensitive and developmentally appropriate strategies to reduce HIV risk-associated sexual behaviors among African American and Latino populations. Dr. Jemmott has directed multiple HIV risk-reduction research projects and has published extensively in the areas of HIV/AIDS prevention and adolescent sexual behavior. She has received many awards for her research and community efforts, including the Congressional Merit Recognition Award, the Outstanding Research Award from the Northern New Jersey Black Nurses Association, and the Governor of New Jersey's Nurse Merit Award in Advanced Nurse Practice. She is a fellow in the American Academy of Nursing and a member of the National Institute of Nursing Research's Advisory Council and the Institute of Medicine.

EDWARD H. KAPLAN, Ph.D., is the William N. and Marie A. Beach Professor of Management Sciences at the Yale School of Management, Professor of Public Health at the Yale School of Medicine, and Director of the Law, Policy and Ethics Core at Yale's Center for Interdisciplinary Research on AIDS. Professor Kaplan received his three master's degrees (in Operations Research, City Planning, and Statistics) and his Doctorate in Urban Studies from the Massachusetts Institute of Technology. Professor Kaplan is an expert in operations research and statistics and has developed novel methods for quantitatively evaluating HIV intervention programs. His current research links the operations of HIV prevention programs to epidemic outcomes, examines the cost-effectiveness of individual intervention programs, and proposes approaches to allocating HIV prevention resources. His past research demonstrating the effectiveness of New Haven's needle exchange program remains among the most creative and important examples of HIV program evaluation to date. He has authored more than 80 peer-reviewed publications and coedited the book *Modeling the AIDS Epidemic: Planning, Policy and Prediction.* For his applications of mathematical and statistical modeling to the study of HIV prevention, he was awarded the 1992 Franz Edelman Management Science Achievement Award, the 1994 Lanchester Prize for the best work in the operations research field, and in 2000 was inducted into the Omega Rho Operations Research Honor Society as an honorary member. Professor Kaplan was twice awarded the Lady Davis Visiting Professorship at the

Hebrew University of Jerusalem where he studied AIDS policy issues facing the State of Israel. Professor Kaplan serves on the editorial boards of the *Journal of AIDS, Health Care Management Science, Journal of Mathematics Applied to Medicine and Biology,* and *Operations Research.*

NANCY KASS, Sc.D., is Associate Professor and Director of the Program in Law, Ethics and Health, in the Johns Hopkins School of Public Health. She is also Associate Professor in the Bioethics Institute at The Johns Hopkins University, and a Fellow of the Kennedy Institute of Ethics at Georgetown. Dr. Kass conducts empirical work in bioethics and health policy. She has published extensively in the fields of HIV/AIDS policy, genetics policy, and research ethics, and is coeditor with Ruth Faden of *HIV, AIDS, and Childbearing: Public Policy, Private Lives.* She served as consultant to the President's Advisory Committee on Human Radiation Experiments, as a member of the Institute of Medicine's Committee on Perinatal Transmission of HIV, and is currently working with the National Bioethics Advisory Commission to examine American investigators' experiences working in developing countries. Other current research projects are focused on genetics and privacy; informed consent in early phase cancer trials, end-of-life decision making; and ethics issues arising in international health research. Dr. Kass completed her doctoral training in health policy from the Johns Hopkins School of Public Health, and was awarded a National Research Service Award to complete a postdoctoral fellowship in bioethics at the Kennedy Institute of Ethics, Georgetown University.

MARSHA LILLIE-BLANTON, Dr.P.H., is Vice-President of the Henry J. Kaiser Family Foundation where she directs the Foundation's policy research and grant-making on access to care for vulnerable populations. Prior to joining the Foundation, Dr. Lillie-Blanton served as Associate Director of Health Services Quality and Public Health Issues of the U.S. General Accounting Office. Dr. Lillie-Blanton has over fifteen years of experience in health policy research, including serving formerly as Associate Director of the Kaiser Commission on the Future of Medicaid. From 1990 to 1994, Dr. Lillie-Blanton was assistant professor of health policy and management at The Johns Hopkins University School of Public Health. She currently holds an adjunct faculty position in The Johns Hopkins School of Public Health. Her primary research interests are in the areas of substance abuse programs and policies and minority health. Her efforts in directing the work of eight research teams analyzing data from the National Medical Expenditure Survey resulted in the publication of *Achieving Equitable Access: Studies of Health Care Issues Affecting Hispanics and African Americans.* Dr. Lillie-Blanton is a member of Medicaid Advisory Committee of the D.C. Department of Health, the National Advisory Council for the Agency for Health Care Policy and Research, and an elected member of the National Academy of Social Insurance. Dr. Lillie-Blanton received her master's and doctorate degree from The Johns Hopkins School of Public Health.

MICHAEL MERSON, M.D., is Dean of Public Health and Chairman of the Department of Epidemiology and Public Health, and the Director of the Center for Interdisciplinary Research on AIDS at Yale University. Dr. Merson received his medical degree from the State University of New York Downstate Medical Center. After serving as a medical intern and resident at Johns Hopkins Hospital, he spent three years in the Enteric Diseases Branch at the Centers for Disease Control and Prevention and then served as the Chief Epidemiologist at the Cholera Research Laboratory in Dhaka, Bangladesh. In 1978, he joined the World Health Organization's Diarrheal Disease Control Programme in Geneva, Switzerland and served as Director of that Programme from 1984 until 1990. In 1987, he was also appointed Director of the WHO Acute Respiratory Infections Control Programme. He was appointed as Director in 1990 and later as Executive Director in 1993 of the WHO Global Programme on AIDS, which was responsible for mobilizing and coordinating the global response to the AIDS pandemic. Dr. Merson received two Commendation Medals from the U.S. Public Health Service, the Arthur S. Flemming Award, the Surgeon General's Exemplary Service Medal, and two honorary degrees. He has served on various National Institutes of Health review panels, advisory committees and institutional boards, and has been elected to the Connecticut Academy of Science and Engineering and the American Epidemiological Society.

EDWARD TRAPIDO, Sc.D., is Professor and Vice Chairman in the Department of Epidemiology and Public Health at the University of Miami School of Medicine. He is also an Associate Director of the Sylvester Comprehensive Cancer Center, and Chief of the Division of Cancer Prevention and Control. Dr. Trapido is the Principal Investigator for the Florida Cancer Data System; the Cancer Information Service for Florida, Puerto Rico, and the U.S. Virgin Islands; and the National Hispanic Leadership Initiative on Cancer. He is also Director and Principal Investigator of the Research and Evaluation Coordinating Center for the State of Florida Tobacco Pilot Program. After earning his master's degree in parasitology from the University of North Carolina, Dr. Trapido was an instructor in environmental health and community medicine at New York's Downstate Medical Center. He then received both a Master's and Sc.D. in Epidemiology from Harvard School of Public Health. Prior to coming to

Miami, Dr. Trapido was a staff fellow in the Division of Cancer Etiology at the National Cancer Institute. His research interests are in tobacco prevention programs and their evaluation, and in working with minority and underserved populations in cancer prevention and control.

STEN H. VERMUND, M.D., Ph.D., is Professor of Epidemiology and International Health, Medicine, and Pediatrics and serves both as Director of the Division of Geographic Medicine and Director of the John J. Sparkman Center for International Public Health Education at the University of Alabama at Birmingham. In addition, he is President of the Gorgas Memorial Institute for Tropical and Preventive Medicine, Inc. Dr. Vermund is an infectious disease epidemiologist and pediatrician with substantial research and training experience overseas. He began his career focused on parasitic infections of public health importance in the Caribbean and Central America. In the late 1980s, his work evolved towards the epidemiology of emerging viruses, first as related to immunosuppression-related parasites, cryptosporidiosis and toxoplasmosis, and later related to human papillomavirus (HPV). The expansion of the HIV epidemic led Dr. Vermund to increasingly focus on the epidemiology and control of sexually transmitted diseases, including HIV and HPV-HIV interactions. From 1988 to 1994, Dr. Vermund was chief of the Vaccine Trials and Epidemiology Branch, Division of AIDS, at the National Institute of Allergy and Infectious Diseases, that resulted in two special commendations from the Surgeon General of the U.S. Public Health Service. His work in HIV vaccine clinical trial preparedness led to the 1994 Superior Service Award, the highest civilian honor in the Public Health Service. Dr. Vermund is now engaged in several HIV/AIDS prevention-related initiatives supported by the National Institutes of Health, the Centers for Disease Control and Prevention, the U.S. Agency for International Development, and the Elizabeth Glaser Pediatric AIDS Foundation.

PAUL VOLBERDING, M.D., is Professor of Medicine, Director of the Positive Health Program and Department of Clinical Oncology, and the founding Director of the Center for AIDS Research at the University of California, San Francisco (UCSF). Dr. Volberding received his M.D. from the University of Minnesota, and completed his residency training at the University of Utah Medical Center. He is board certified in internal medicine and oncology. Although an oncologist by training, Dr. Volberding has devoted the majority of his efforts to establishing comprehensive and multidisciplinary systems of care for HIV-infected persons and to conducting clinical investigations of antiretroviral drugs. His particular interests include testing strategies for improving HIV outcomes by optimizing the timing and choice of therapy. As the codirector of the UCSF Center for AIDS Research, he facilitates and conducts translational research crossing the boundaries of basic, clinical, and behavioral sciences. Dr. Volberding also directs a comprehensive HIV-focused website (HIVInSite) and chairs a nonprofit educational organization, International AIDS Society-USA. Dr. Volberding is a member of the Institute of Medicine and has served on several committees addressing HIV/AIDS issues.

ANDREW ZOLOPA, M.D., is Assistant Professor of Medicine at the Stanford University School of Medicine. He is also the Director of the Stanford Positive Care Program, the Chief of the AIDS Medicine Division at Santa Clara Valley Medical Center. Dr. Zolopa received his M.D. from the University of California at Los Angeles School of Medicine, was a Robert Wood Johnson Clinical Scholar, and completed a Postdoctoral Fellowship in Infectious Diseases and Geographic Medicine at the Stanford University Medical Center. He is board certified in infectious diseases and maintains an active HIV clinical practice at Stanford University Medical Center. Dr. Zolopa's past research includes population-based studies of HIV and TB prevalence and risk factors in homeless populations. This work has led to ongoing studies of HIV treatment, adherence to antiretrovirals, and drug resistance in inner-city urban populations in which he collaborates. Since 1996, Dr. Zolopa has been actively involved in clinical investigation with a particular focus on the role of HIV-1 resistance testing in treatment. He is a Co-Investigator with Stanford University's AIDS Clinical trials Group (ACTG) and is the Co-Founder of the Clinic-based Investigator's group (CBIG)—a national multi-center group evaluating the effectiveness and safety of antiretroviral therapies through observational cohort studies.

Expert Consultants

IVAN JUZANG, M.B.A., is founder and President of MEE Productions, Inc. Since 1990, MEE has provided communication research, media production, and marketing services to both private and public sector clients in the United States and abroad. Mr. Juzang manages and produces all of MEE's research-based communication projects targeting African Americans and urban youth, and designs and directs MEE's urban marketing campaigns and community teams. He has moderated hundreds of MEE focus groups and has been a primary researcher in all of MEE's national studies. MEE first received prominence with the release of its primary research study funded by funded by The Robert Wood Johnson Foundation, entitled The MEE Report: "Reaching the Hip-Hop Generation," which identified effective communication strategies to encourage prosocial behavior among inner-city teenagers around alcohol and tobacco prevention. Currently, Mr. Juzang serves as a board member of the Alan Guttmacher Institute. Mr. Juzang was also an Adjunct Professor at Temple University's School of Communications, Department of Broadcasting Telecommunications and Mass Media. Mr. Juzang received his M.B.A. from the Wharton School of Business.

MICHAEL A. STOTO, Ph.D., is Professor and Chair of the Department of Epidemiology and Biostatistics at the George Washington University School of Public Health and Health Services. Dr. Stoto received an A.B. in Statistics from Princeton University, and an A.M. and Ph.D. in Statistics from Harvard University in 1979. He was an Associate Professor of Public Policy at Harvard's John F. Kennedy School of Government, and is an Adjunct Professor of Biostatistics in the Harvard School of Public Health. From 1987 through 1998, Dr. Stoto served as a Senior Staff Officer and Director of the Division of Health Promotion and Disease Prevention of the Institute of Medicine, National Academy of Sciences. He is currently a consultant to the IOM on a variety of public health issues. Dr. Stoto's research and teaching interests include a variety of topics related to the use of statistical data and quantitative analysis in public health policy. His research interests include methodological topics in epidemiology, biostatistics, and demography, as well as substantive issues in public health policy and practice. He also has strong interests in research synthesis and meta-analysis, community health assessment, risk analysis and management, and the evaluation of public health interventions. At the Institute of Medicine, Dr. Stoto was responsible for projects in occupational and environmental health (including *Veterans and Agent Orange*), HIV/AIDS (such as *HIV and the Blood Supply*), maternal and child health (including *Reducing the Odds: Preventing Perinatal Transmission of HIV in the United States*) and public health practice (such as *Healthy Communities* and *Improving Health in the Community*).

Liaisons from the Board on Health Promotion and Disease Prevention

JOYCE SEIKO KOBAYASHI, M.D., is currently Director of the HIV/AIDS Neuropsychiatric Consultation Service at Denver Health Medical Center, Associate Professor in the Department of Psychiatry at the University of Colorado Health Sciences Center, and Associate Faculty member of the Department of Healthcare Ethics, Humanities and the Law there. Dr. Kobayashi received her undergraduate training at Stanford University, her M.D. from the University of Rochester School of Medicine, and completed her psychiatric training at Albert Einstein College of Medicine. She completed a subspecialty fellowship in Consultation/Liaison Psychiatry through Mt. Sinai College of Medicine, and has since specialized in the psychiatric treatment of people with HIV/AIDS. She was an American Psychiatric Association / National Institute of Mental Health (APA/NIMH) Minority Fellow and has served on a number of national Committees and Councils of the APA. During her tenure as Chairperson of the APA Committee of Asian American Psychiatrists, she organized the first International Symposium on Psychiatric Research in Asia. She has served for many years as a member of the National Commission on AIDS of the APA, where she was one of the authors of the needle exchange policy for the Association. She served as a national examiner for the Board of Psychiatry and Neurology. She has been the recipient of several awards, including the Dinkelspiel Award at Stanford, Colorado Woman of the Year in Health and Human Services from the Colorado Asian Pacific Women's Network, and Rocky Mountain Regional AIDS Conference Award for Service to People with AIDS. Dr. Kobayashi has published a variety of articles and chapters on HIV/AIDS, biomedical ethics, women's issues, transcultural psychiatry and has given invited lectures at regional and national AIDS meetings.

KATHLEEN E. TOOMEY, M.D., M.P.H., is Director of the Division of Public Health, Georgia Department of Human Resources. Dr. Toomey received her M.D. and M.P.H. degrees from Harvard Medical School and Harvard School of Public Health. After completing a residency in family medicine at the University of Washington in Seattle, she served as clinical director of the Kotzebue Service Unit with the Indian Health Service in Northwest Alaska. She was then selected as a Pew Health Policy Research Fellow at the University of California, San Francisco, Institute for Health Policy Studies, where she worked under former Assistant Secretary for Health, Dr. Philip R. Lee. She later held a number of positions in the Division of STD/HIV Prevention at the Centers for Disease Control and Prevention including EIS officer and Associate Director. She then served as a legislative assistant on health issues for U.S. Senator John Chafee (R-RI). She received the CDC Award for Contributions to the Advancement of Women and the Public Health Service Plaque for Outstanding Leadership. Dr. Toomey has served on the boards of many professional and national organizations, including the American Public Health Association and the Alan Guttmacher Institute. She currently chairs the Public Health Committee of the Georgia Academy of Family Physicians and serves on the Public Health and Preventive Medicine Committee of the Medical Association of Georgia. Dr. Toomey holds faculty appointments at the Rollins School of Public Health, Emory University, Emory School of Medicine, and Morehouse University School of Medicine. Her research interests include women's health and reproductive health policy, health services in underserved areas, and the epidemiology and prevention of STDs and HIV/AIDS.

Staff

MONICA S. RUIZ, Ph.D., M.P.H. is a Senior Program Officer at the Institute of Medicine and the Study Director for the Committee on HIV Prevention Strategies. Prior to joining the IOM in 1999, she was a Research Associate at the University of Connecticut, where she worked with colleagues at the Yale AIDS Program in developing a clinician-delivered prevention intervention for HIV-infected persons in outpatient care. In 1998, Dr. Ruiz served as the Counseling and Social Support Advisor for the Joint United Nations Programme on HIV/AIDS (UNAIDS) in Geneva, Switzerland; while in that post, she also served as the UNAIDS liaison to The Voluntary HIV Counseling and Testing Efficacy Study. Dr. Ruiz received her doctorate in Preventive Medicine from the University of Southern California School of Medicine, and her Masters degree in Public Health from the University of California, Berkeley. She also completed a post-doctoral fellowship with the Center for AIDS Prevention Studies at the University of California, San Francisco.

ALICIA R. GABLE, M.P.H., is a Research Associate for the Institute of Medicine's Committee on HIV Prevention Strategies. Prior to joining the IOM's Division of Health Promotion and Disease Prevention in 1999, Ms. Gable completed a fellowship in health services administration at the Washington Hospital Center in Washington, DC. Ms. Gable also worked as an economist at Research Triangle Institute and Triangle Economic Research in Durham, NC, where she conducted several health valuation surveys and natural resource damage assessment studies. Ms. Gable holds an M.P.H. in health management and policy from the University of Michigan at Ann Arbor and a B.A. in economics and international studies from the University of North Carolina at Chapel Hill.

ROSE MARIE MARTINEZ, Sc.D., is the Director of the Institute of Medicine's (IOM) Board on Health Promotion and Disease Prevention. Prior to joining the IOM, she was a Senior Health Researcher at Mathematica Policy Research where she conducted research on the impact of health system change on the public health infrastructure, access to care for vulnerable populations, managed care, and the health care workforce. Dr. Martinez is a former Assistant Director for Health Financing and Policy with the U.S. General Accounting Office where she directed evaluations and policy analysis in the area of national and public health issues. Dr. Martinez received her doctorate from the Johns Hopkins School of Hygiene and Public Health.

DONNA ALMARIO is the research assistant for the Institute of Medicine's (IOM) Committee on HIV Prevention Strategies. Ms. Almario joined the IOM's Division of Health Promotion and Disease Prevention in 1997 and has worked on other IOM studies including, *Reducing the Odds: Preventing Perinatal Transmission of HIV in the United States* and *Ending Neglect: Eliminating Tuberculosis in the United States*. Prior to joining the IOM, she worked at Georgetown University Medical Center's Lombardi Cancer Center. Ms. Almario graduated from Vassar College with a bio-psychology degree and is presently working towards a masters in public health degree at the George Washington University's School of Public Health and Health Services.

ANNA STATON is the project assistant for the Institute of Medicine's (IOM) Committee on HIV Prevention Strategies. Ms. Staton joined the IOM's Division of Health Promotion and Disease Prevention in 1999. Prior to joining the IOM, she worked at the Baltimore Women's Health Study. Ms. Staton graduated from the University of Maryland Baltimore County with a visual arts (major) and women's studies (minor) degree. She is currently working toward a masters in public administration degree at George Washington University's School of Business and Public Management.

Index

A

Abstinence education programs, components of, 119n

"Abstinence-plus" programs, 117

Access
to drug abuse treatment, 106-116
to sterile drug injection equipment, 114-116

ACHSP. *See* Advisory Committee for HIV and STD Prevention

Acquired immunodeficiency syndrome. *See* AIDS

ACSUS. *See* AIDS Cost and Services Utilization Survey

ADAMHA Reorganization Act of 1992, 167

ADAP. *See* AIDS Drug Assistance Program

Adolescent AIDS cases, by exposure category, 141

Adolescent Family Life Act (AFLA), 118-119

Adolescent sex workers, 189

Adult AIDS cases, by exposure category, 141

Adult correctional systems, HIV/AIDS education, harm reduction, and discharge planning programs in U.S., 122

Advisory Committee for HIV and STD Prevention (ACHSP), 74

AFLA. *See* Adolescent Family Life Act

Africa, HIV incidence in, 105, 140

African Americans
Medicaid services provided to, 57
rates of AIDS infection among, 143-145

Agency for Health Care Quality and Research, spending on HIV/AIDS, 172

Aggregate HIV incidence, estimating, 173

AIDS cases
adult/adolescent, by exposure category, 141
and co-occurring conditions, 147-148, 152
geographic distribution of, 145-146
inadequacy of reporting based on, 15
increases in, 1
lag in diagnosis time for, 4, 81n
perinatally acquired, 144-145
providers caring for, 55-56
"public health" responses to, 22
in racial and ethnic minorities, 144-145
rates per 100,000 population, 146
and sexual orientation, 2
in women, 142-143
in youth, 143-144